Ageless Aging

Ageless Aging

HOW SCIENCE IS WINNING
THE BATTLE TO HELP YOU
EXTEND YOUR HEALTHY AND
PRODUCTIVE YEARS

Ruth Winter

CROWN PUBLISHERS, INC.
NEW YORK

TO
Robin, Craig, and Grant
WHO

CONTRIBUTED

APPRECIABLY

TO MY

AGING

Library of Congress Catalog Card Number: 72-96640
ISBN: 0-517-505762

Printed in the United States of America

Published simultaneously in Canada by General Publishing
Company Limited

Contents

Acknowledgments

THE AUTHOR WISHES TO thank Nathan Shock, Ph.D., Chief of the National Institutes of Health Gerontology Research Center; Charles Barrows, Ph.D., Chief of the Gerontology Center's Section on Environment and Genetics; Ewald Busse, M.D., Chairman of the Department of Psychiatry at Duke University Medical School and first Director of its Aging Research Center; Thomas Hodge McGavack, M.D., of Martinsburg, West Virginia; Arthur Winter, M.D., of East Orange, New Jersy; and James Hamilton, Ph.D., Professor of Anatomy, Downstate Medical Center, New York University College of Medicine, who not only took time from their busy schedules for interviews, but also checked the appropriate chapters for accuracy. The author also wishes to thank the many others whose contributions made this book possible, including Denham Harman, M.D., Professor of Medicine at the University of Nebraska; Edward Henderson, M.D., President of the Aging Research Foundation; Erdman Palmore, Ph.D., Associate Professor of Medical Sociology, Duke University Medical Center; Herbert Kupperman, M.D., Associate Professor of Medicine, New York University College of Medicine; Frank Chappell, Director of Science Information, American Medical Association; Dan Rogers, Public Information Officer, NIH Gerontology Research Center; and Vance Whitfield, Assistant Public Relations Director, Duke University Medical Center. A special thanks is due to my editor, Paul Nadan, without whose skill and encouragement this book could not have been completed.

Chapter 1

How Long Would You Like to Live?

How LONG WOULD YOU like to live? A hundred years? A thousand years? Indefinitely?

Before you answer that, don't picture yourself wrinkled, incapacitated, unemployed, and unwanted. Picture yourself as you would be at twenty-five years with full adult vigor, appearance, and capability.

Eternal youth, that elusive goal that humans have sought since they first realized that they withered with the passage of time, is in sight. Gerontologists, scientists who are devoting their careers to the study of the aging process, believe they have some of the answers to why and how we age and that mankind is on the brink of being able to slow, arrest, and perhaps even reverse the aging process.

Impossible? Who would have thought it possible thirty years ago that tuberculosis or pneumonia could be cured by pills, and who really believed that men could walk on the moon?

The fact is that no one has ever really died of old age. A death officially listed as "old age" a century ago in a Massachusetts hospital was for a woman forty-five years old.

Lord Byron, feeling the burden of old age, wrote on his birthday:

> "My days are in the yellow leaf;
> The flowers and fruits of love are gone;
> The worm, the canker, and the grief
> Are mine alone!"

1

He was thirty-six.

What we consider aging—wrinkled skin, hardening of the arteries, gray hair, deafness, frail bones—can be found in small children. Such signs of aging are symptoms of disease. If one conclusion has been reached from gerontological research, it is that disease is one thing and aging quite another.

There is something about aging, of course, that makes us more susceptible to disease. For instance, when pneumonia strikes at twenty years of age, our chances of dying from it are two per one hundred thousand. When it strikes at eighty-five years, our chances are increased to about one thousand per one hundred thousand.

But if we had through life the same resistance to stress and disease that we had at twenty, it is estimated that more than half of us would live seven hundred years or more.

Theoretically, the human body should live forever since it is a self-repairing organism. We should go on indefinitely until, by choice or accident, we die.

In practice, however, infinite life is beyond us, but we have made great progress keeping humans alive for longer periods.

At the beginning of recorded history, longevity averaged eighteen years. In 1900 the average life-span was forty-five years, and by the mid-1950s it was seventy years. In 1900 only one out of ten Americans could expect to reach sixty-five years. Today, two out of three celebrate their sixty-fifth birthday.

Presumably, our ancestors who lived until eighteen years and those who survived to forty-five years started out with the same basic equipment as we did. They didn't live as long because they lacked the environmental protection and medical care we receive.

The great historical physicians Hippocrates and Maimonides probably would not have believed one country would have 28 million humans over sixty-five years of age. Yet, in only eight years the United States will have that many and they will be nearly 10 percent of the population. A century ago there were just over a million over sixty-five and they made up approximately 3 percent of the population. By the year 2000 government estimates predict 30 million Americans sixty-five years or older; of these, 13 million will be over seventy-five years old. We will then have as many citizens over seventy-five as we had over sixty-five in 1950. The 1970 census reported 106,441 Americans over one hundred years, and the 1971 Social Security rolls had 5,253 people past the century mark.

But having many people over sixty-five or seventy-five or one hundred is not a goal in itself. They must be "living," not merely "existing." Many of our sixty-five-year-olds are physically equal to their fifty-year-old counterparts at the turn of the century. The oldest American on the Social Security rolls, Charlie Smith, age 130, runs a small candy shop in Bartow, a rural village about midway between Tampa and Lake Wales, Florida. Charlie was born in Liberia, Africa, July 4, 1842. This was documented in 1854 when, at the age of twelve, he was sold at a New Orleans slave auction to a Texas rancher and again when he applied for Social Security. He was just twenty-one when the Emancipation Proclamation was signed by President Lincoln, and 113 when he retired from his work as a fruit picker in Florida. His employer felt that Charlie was "getting too old" to climb trees.

The Russians claim 47 times more centenarians per million residents than we do, 86 times more than France, 102 times more than Britain, and 610 times more than Japan. Their oldest citizen is 168-year-old Shirali Mislimov, from the village of Barzavu, in Azerbaijan. He was born in 1805 and, according to the Soviets, "feels fine. He enjoys riding and gardening. A deputy to the Village Soviet [a member of the local governing body], he ably discharges his duties of a people's representative. The oldest man in this country has a very good nature. He never gets angry and only laughs merrily at the mischief of his great-grandchildren and his great-great grandchildren. His pulse is normal—72 beats a minute. His blood pressure is that of a healthy young man and his weight is 62 kg [136 pounds]."

The Russians report four times more long-lived persons in the mountainous regions of Dagestan than on the plains. In the Bumbet and Tlyarata mountainous districts, nearly one hundred of every ten thousand residents is over one hundred years. Over 60 percent of the Georgians work past age eighty on farms. They hunt, ride, and generally live as they did long ago.

Reaching extreme old age is not because of something one does. It is more because of something one doesn't do. It's a matter of not succumbing to childhood diseases or to other infections.

Even if there were a cure or a preventative for all major diseases, how much longer could we live? The most that could be achieved by further disease-oriented biomedical research thus far is about fifteen additional years. If the number one killer—cardiovascular disease—were eliminated, life expectancy would be increased by only ten years. If cancer were eliminated, it would increase longevity by 2.5 years.

What is needed to greatly prolong our lives is a basic understanding of why and how we age, and then the chemicals that will combat or prevent that process of deterioration. These chemicals may be entirely new compounds or they may already be in limited use today. To be truly beneficial, however, they must be inexpensive, widely available, and without serious side effects.

With computer capability and advances in chemical analysis, it should be feasible to analyze what is missing chemically in a sixty-year-old that was present at twenty years, and then replace those missing elements.

The Rand Corporation, which specializes in anticipating breakthroughs in various aspects of technology and science, predicts the chemical control of aging by the year 2025, with artificial organs made of plastic and electronic components available by 1990; biochemicals to stimulate the growth of new organs and limbs are predicted by 2020.

We needn't wait that long. There are many things that

we can do right now, thanks to science, to increase our vigor and prolong youthfulness. These follow in subsequent chapters.

The always conservative American Medical Association's Council on Medical Services maintains that with intelligent application of existing knowledge, we should all live to be ninety to one hundred or more years. The AMA advises that children should be trained right now to meet the probability that most of them will live past ninety, and many beyond one hundred years.

How long is the ultimate human life-span? It could be as varied as the life-span between species and among the same species. Some plants are annuals and do not survive the first winter, while the giant sequoia tree lives 3,000 years and the bristle cone pine 4,600 years. The dog who suffers all the same ills as the human, including heart disease, diabetes, and cancer, lives twelve to eighteen years compared to the human life-span of seventy to one hundred years. The species closest, physiologically, to humans are chimpanzees, gorillas, and gibbons, who live from thirty to forty years. A Galapagos tortoise lives two hundred years or more. In some human families death cuts off the generation in the forties, while in others all live to ninety and beyond.

Some gerontologists opt for about 120 years as the ultimate life-span. Others are convinced it is infinite.

The English author Jonathan Swift really summed it up when he said, "Every man desires to live long, but no man would be old."

In the not too distant future that desire may be answered. We will have ageless aging.

Chapter 2

How Old Are You?

EVEN IF YOU KNOW the exact minute, hour, day, and year of your birth, you can't answer that question because you are really made up of three ages:

- Your chronological age marked by the calendar.
- Your physiological, or biological, age—the most important because it encompasses the elemental stuff with which you were born and is influenced by heredity and environment. Furthermore, your various organs may be different biological ages. Your heart, for instance, may be thirty years old, but your liver sixty years.
- Your psychological age, which is nearly as important. In fact, as one government researcher summed it up, "Aging is a matter of mind over matter—if you don't mind, it doesn't matter."

Of course, we all mind aging. That is, we mind losing what we associate with youth—beauty, sexual attractiveness, health, strength, employment, anticipation of the future, and a sense of usefulness.

And yet, in certain civilizations, the older a person is, the more valued. And we will see in a later chapter that even sexual functioning can be maintained in extreme old age.

What we call aging is not the same for everyone. We all know people of forty years who are old and people of eighty years who are young. In fact, gerontologists cannot examine a person whose age is unknown and with any assurance determine that the person is thirty years or fifty years or sixty years. They may miss by as much as fifteen years.

There are certain clues, of course, to how old you really are. If you are a redhead or a blue-eyed blond, your skin will develop wrinkles faster than a brunette's.

If your blood pressure or serum cholesterol greatly exceeds normal, you may be physically seven, fifteen, or even twenty years older than your contemporaries.

If you had four grandparents who lived to be eighty, you are probably four years younger than your less fortunate friends. If you are a man whose father died at age eighty or more, you have the best life expectancy. In fact, you will live almost ten years longer than a man whose father died under fifty years of age.

Do you live in the country? If so, you will probably survive five years longer than if you lived in the city. If you make your home in Alaska, your chances of premature death are the lowest in the United States—4.7 compared to Washington, D.C., where the death rate is the highest in the United States, 13.3. Ironically, Alaska has the lowest percentage of MDs per population in the country, while Washington, D.C., has the highest.

If you are a Norwegian male, you will live an average of two years longer than your American counterpart. If you are a Canadian female, you will survive two years longer than your American cousins.

If you smoke, your lungs may be ten years older than your chronological age. Even if both your parents lived beyond eighty years, you will die younger than nonsmoking offspring of long-lived parents. And it may not be just from the physical damage of cigarette smoke. Studies show that smokers are more rebellious than nonsmokers.

The statistics mentioned above really demonstrate that your biological age depends on where you live, how you live, and the basic equipment you inherited from your parents. These figures, of course, give the odds based on averages.

A 103-year-old man being interviewed by a newspaper

reporter summed it up well. The reporter, marveling at the man's advanced age, asked:

"If you had your life to live over again, would you do anything differently?"

"Well," the old man said as he sipped straight bourbon from a glass, "if I'd known that I was going to live to be 103, I sure would have taken better care of myself."

Theoretically, your body should take care of itself. It has enormous capacity. In approximately seventy years of life, you will eat fourteen hundred times your body weight and spend five full years just putting food into your mouth. Every year your heart beats about 36,792,000 times, you breathe 8,409,600 times, and you move 750 major muscles ad infinitum.

Your body can take extreme punishment and still function. You can get along without your bladder, gall bladder, spleen, or appendix. You can lose a kidney, a lung, quarts of blood, your pituitary gland, half your brain, both your eyes, all your teeth. In fact, you can live with just half a body as long as it is from the waist up.

Why does this magnificent machine wear down, especially in view of the fact that it is self-repairing? Why does it wear down at a different rate from one person to another, although both start out with seemingly the same equipment?

When does aging begin?

Physically, most humans mature at about twenty-five to thirty years of age. This is the period when the body's framework reaches its maximum size and strength. It is at this point that we begin to age. But aging starts also at the moment of fertilization, even though at first such aging is positive because the body grows and develops.

In a study of more than five hundred aortas (the major artery carrying blood from the heart), fat deposits that lead to hardening of the arteries and age-associated diseases such as strokes and senility were found in all individuals three years of age and over. All those of eighteen years had fibrous plaques, which impede the proper functioning of the arteries.

Blood vessels collected from patients with and without

poor circulation in the fingers and toes showed no perfect fingertip vessels for any of them over fourteen years.

Examples of early aging are numerous. For instance, when babies no longer need their small, fragile milk teeth, they begin to lose them around six years. Their teeth "age" and fall out and are replaced by stronger, more deep-rooted teeth. But, over 50 percent of us have at least one cavity in our teeth by the age of two years. Gum irritation is present in four out of five in the twelve- to fourteen-year-age group, and peridontal disease occurs in 4 percent of those between the ages of thirteen and fifteen. On the average, a twenty-one-year-old has five teeth missing.

Yet, such early problems as hardening of the arteries and missing teeth are merely symptoms that we associate with aging. But can both be prevented?

There are at least five types of hyperlipemia, an over-abundance of fats in the blood that may lead to clogging and hardening of the arteries. In turn, this leads to such problems associated with "aging" as strokes, senility, heart attacks, and insufficient blood to nourish the extremities. These fats are primarily made up of cholesterol and triglycerides, saturated fats. Saturated fats are solid at room temperature and are usually derived from animals. Unsaturated fats are liquid at room temperature and most often derive from vegetables. The fat from a piece of beef would be a saturated fat, and the oil from the safflower would be an unsaturated fat.

By manipulating the diet and making it low in saturated fats and in sugar, doctors have been able to lower considerably the amount of saturated fats in the blood serum, and, according to some studies, prolong the lives of former heart attack victims following this diet regime. Although such results are still controversial, no one can argue the fact that in populations that eat a low-saturated fat diet and a low sugar diet, hardening of the arteries is practically nonexistent. On the other hand, there are people who eat a diet high in saturated fats who also do not suffer from artery ills.

Nevertheless, people who maintain a low fat, low sugar diet, and who do not smoke and who do not have high blood pressure, will greatly reduce the likelihood of developing the age-associated artery diseases. Thanks to modern medicines, most blood pressure problems can be kept in control.

For those of us with already clogged arteries and high blood fat levels, it is possible to lower those levels chemically, just as it is possible to lower blood pressure. A drug, clofibrate, reduces serum cholesterol from 7 to 35 percent and triglycerides from 20 to 60 percent. Clofibrate, it has been reported, is even capable of somewhat reversing the process of already clogged arteries, but whether it will greatly prolong life or be used as a preventative is yet to be determined. What is proved is that it is possible chemically to treat this symptom of aging. And if clofibrate isn't able to do the entire job, an improved drug probably can.

Tooth loss can be prevented. There are simple and effective methods. Improved oral hygiene alone will bring about improved oral periodontal health, whereas cessation of good oral hygiene in a healthy mouth will lead to discernible inflammation of the gums in from ten to twenty-one days. The principal pathologic disease leading to tooth loss from gingival disease is inflammation.

That old, mundane object, the toothbrush, is a critical item. In no other field of medicine is there a device that a patient may use to prevent a disease as effectively as the toothbrush. Furthermore, fluoridation of the water and application of fluorides or sealants to the surface of the teeth, and the use of dental floss have all proved tooth decay and tooth loss can be prevented.

If aging of tissues is to be prevented, we must understand these tissues at least as well as we understand arteries and teeth. We must find out how they deteriorate and why.

Previously held ideas are being repudiated. For instance, standards of normality in the past have always been measured by testing healthy young medical students. However, what is "normal" for a twenty-year-old is apparently not "normal" for a seventy-year-old. Take the glucose tolerance test, for example. Using standards of blood sugar set for young people, nearly half of the nondiabetic old subjects tested would be labeled diabetic. Yet, it was discovered that the older subjects were not diabetic. It just takes a longer time for their blood sugar levels to return to normal after they receive a test dose of sugar. The diabetic's blood sugar never does return to normal levels.

On the other hand, some ninety-year-olds have the same amount of healthy blood flow through their kidneys as have twenty-year-olds; instead of deteriorating mentally, some fifty-year-olds actually do better on intelligence tests than they did in college. Experience and emotional maturity plus unknown factors may contribute to such improvements.

New findings indicate only how much more we need to know about the aging process. For instance, we now know that blood flow to the brain is nearly the same throughout life. Nerve fibers connecting directly with the muscles show little impairment with age and yet impulses sent by nerves slow from 140 miles an hour in youth to 110 miles an hour in age. Why?

Under resting, nonstressful conditions, there is little measurable variation in the chemical composition of the blood between the healthy twenty-year-old and the healthy seventy-year-old. Yet, put them both under physical or mental stress, and the twenty-year-old will outperform the seventy-year-old. The ability to withstand physical stress fades pretty rapidly. Swimmers, for instance, are old in their twenties and boxers are elderly at thirty years.

The various measurements by themselves do not mean much, but when they are put together they begin to give clues about how and why we age.

Take the lungs, for instance. The oxygen the blood takes up from the lungs and transports to the tissues during exercise falls substantially with age; the blood of a twenty-year-old man can take up, on the average, almost four liters of oxygen per minute; the blood of a seventy-five-year-old man can take up only 1.5 liters per minute. If a man were not exposed to lung disease, pollution, cigarette smoke, and other noxious inhalants, would his lungs at seventy-five years take up the same amount of oxygen as a twenty-year-old man? Would he still have "young" lungs?

The same holds true for the kidney. The amount of blood flow through the kidneys shows a decrease between 6 and 10 percent every decade. In other words, the kidney flow in an eighty-year-old man is about half that in the twenty- to thirty-year-old man. Is this due to damage or to aging?

The average man's work rate between thirty and seventy-five years declines 40 percent; his handgrip 45 percent, and his taste and sensitivity 64 percent. A man of sixty years running for a streetcar has a harder time catching it than a twenty-year-old. Yet, in measuring the individual components, like certain muscle groups, one can find very little difference between the twenty-year-old and the sixty-year-old.

In norms of hearing and in blood and dental measurements, men age more quickly than women—until the age of fifty years. From thirty on, Negro males are an average of five years older than white males of the same chronological age. Women appear to age fastest in their forties—twenty-three years of aging in ten calendar years

Obviously, there are usually vast differences in physical performance and health between the young and old. These changes are being recorded and averaged. But are such changes really due to aging? If so, they would be common to all.

If in a study of elderly volunteers, twenty-seven out of seven hundred had no hardening of the arteries and their blood pressure and blood chemistry were almost exactly the same as much younger persons', then who really were normal? The 673 who had hardening of the arteries so commonly seen in the elderly or the 27 whose blood vessels had escaped the so-called symptom of aging?

Blood pressure does not necessarily rise with age, although so many older people do have high blood pressure. In a study, many men between the ages of twenty-four and fifty-four years had no rise at all. But those who did have high blood pressure at the age of fifty-four developed it by the age of thirty-four years, the result not of "normal" aging but of disease.

Are the familiar alterations that we all have observed in ourselves and others normal or symptoms of disease? Why do they occur at different times in members of the same human species? Why do they not occur at all in some people?

When we examine the process of aging, we must remember that no matter how old we are, we all have cells in our bodies that are only a few hours or a few days old. These cells are not aged, although the rest of us may be.

How old are you? You are as old as your oldest vital organ, which may be younger than your chronological age or many years older. How old you feel and act depends not only on your biological age but upon that immeasurable component that makes life interesting.

Chapter 3

The Secret of Eternal Youth Is in a Single Cell

WITHIN THE HEART OF every human cell there is an awesome chemical that holds sway over life and death, physical disease and health, intelligence, beauty, growth, and aging. It is DNA, a deoxyribonucleic acid, the code of life. It is contained in a gene within a nucleus less than three-thousandths of an inch wide.

Each cell's DNA has the information and capability to organize the billions and trillions of cells that make you an individual unlike any other on earth. Each cell's DNA also has the power to suppress actions. The fertilized human egg cell, for instance, has all the information for growing hair, but doesn't grow hair. It could also become muscle, brain, bone, kidney, and all the other construction materials that go into building a human being. Only as the original egg cell divides and multiplies, do some of its descendants become hair cells, and others become brain cells, bone cells, and so forth.

When the living human body is completed, it is made up of basically two types of cells—those that continue to divide and those that do not. Skin, blood, and liver cells, for instance, divide at varying rates. Each cell splits and reduplicates itself. Nerve, brain, and muscle cells do not divide. Once you obtain your full quota, that's it. If you lose one, it's gone for good.

The aging of the body is believed to be caused by the loss of cells and the decline in the ability of the remaining cells to function.

The human body loses from 1 to 2 percent of its cells through death each day. It is estimated that your weight would double every fifty to one hundred days if such cells did not die and you continued to make new ones.

For example, every twelve to fourteen days a skin cell of the forearm will move from its newly dividing state to its death at the outermost dead layer of skin. A liver cell, on the other hand, dies in about ten months. This adds up to millions of dead cells each day.

Organs that have cells that divide frequently do not age as rapidly as organs equipped with nondividing cells. The reason is that nondividing cells cannot readily overcome damage to their DNA mutations. Cells that divide have a chance to get rid of faulty DNA and thereby do not perpetuate the damage or cause aging. The damaged cell will usually die right away or lose out in competition with normal neighbors and be replaced with a healthy one.

Because muscle, nerve, and brain cells do not divide, it is not surprising that muscle weakness and memory difficulty are among two of the earliest signs of aging.

Each cell, whether it is the type that divides or not, is programmed for a certain life-span. It has been demonstrated in the laboratory that under the very best of environmental conditions, fibroplasts—cells of the connective tissue—will divide about fifty times and then die, presumably living out their lifetime as they would have in their original host.

The program-making of each cell, and consequently of each human being, is comparable to a movie film. All the action, the events, are prerecorded on the film. How long the film runs depends on how fast it runs through the projector. It can be speeded up and, therefore, finished in a shorter period of time. It can be cut off in the middle and never finished. However, from birth, the entire footage of the film is preset. The length of each person's film footage depends on what he inherited from his parents, the genetic DNA in the cell. The time it takes to play depends not only on inheritance but on environmental factors.

It is possible that none of us ever uses his full footage of film, and that we all die before our time.

Premature death can be demonstrated with a single cell. Take a young fibroplast cell and put it in a laboratory dish with the serum from an old animal. As described before, fibroplast cells will divide fifty times under optimum conditions. But under conditions in which the serum containing a young fibroplast is from an old animal, the young cell will not develop and divide. Something missing from the serum of old animals will not permit the young cell to live out its preset program of dividing fifty times.

No cell lives forever. How does a cell die?

There are many theories, some backed by impressive experimental evidence about what happens to the cell to cause it to age.

Take the radiation theory. A combination physiologist-physicist, Dr. Howard Curtis of Brookhaven Laboratory, was assigned to find out the effect of atomic radiation on living things during World War II. To do so, he exposed mice to various doses of radiation. He noticed that the irradiated mice died of all the same diseases other mice die of, but they did so sooner. They aged and then died prematurely.

Dr. Curtis's observations in mice were later observed in victims of the atomic bomb dropped on Nagasaki, Japan. Those who were exposed to radiation but survived aged prematurely, and developed a high incidence of leukemia, a disease associated with broken chromosomes.

Now, when large doses of radiation occur, the damage is obvious. The pathological changes are directly attributable to cell damage so severe that the cells cannot recover. In chronic, low level radiation, however, the effects are not so clear. We are all exposed to radiation, not only from medical X rays but from rocks, soil, and outer space. This kind of radiation occurs in minute doses and certainly does not produce the dramatic effects of radiation emitted by the atomic and hydrogen bombs.

One of the effects of large amounts of radiation is to damage the cell's code of life—DNA—causing mutation. The theory is that significant amounts of radiation cause premature aging and shorten life by fouling up the normal transmission of DNA information within the nondividing cells, and from generation to generation in the dividing cells. The smaller, everyday doses may do the same thing as larger doses, but take a longer time to do it.

This is an interesting and logical theory but how do you go about proving it?

With a vested interest in the answers, the United States Atomic Energy Commission has been financing studies of the chronic, long term or delayed effects of irradiation in man and animals. Information is being gathered from accidental exposures to radiation; for example, the low level chronic exposure of radiologists during the practice of their profession; the Marshallese people who were exposed to fallout during a weapons test in the Pacific Ocean in 1954 and workers involved in radiation accidents.

In the 1930s it was observed that radiologists died at an average age of 55.8 years, five years earlier than the general population. By the 1960s, when the physicians had learned to better protect themselves against radiation, their average age at death was 70.1 However, in the 1930s and the 1960s radiologists had a higher death rate from leukemia than the general population. Otherwise, they died from the same things that everyone else did. In other words, there was a nonspecific but definite life-shortening effect upon radiologists from their exposure to radiation. As they better protected themselves from radiation, they lived longer.

Among the Marshallese, the most significant finding of their exposure to radiation was the development of thyroid gland abnormalities. Most of the abnormalities were discovered in children who were less than ten years old when exposed. No such abnormalities were found in children not exposed. In addition to the thyroid problems and some impairment of growth in children exposed, there were slightly reduced levels of certain blood elements during the first ten years after exposure in the Marshallese, a possible increase in miscarriages among exposed women during the first four years after the accident, and an increase in the incidence of moles on skin areas that had been the sites of burns from beta radiation in fallout particles that had adhered to the skin.

Yet, unlike the radiologists and the Japanese victims of the atomic bomb, the Marshallese showed no cases of leukemia and no apparent life shortening.

The answer to the paradox may be in the inborn ability of certain genes, perhaps in the Marshallese, to withstand attacks by radiation and other mutagens to their DNA. The influence of heredity on the integrity of the cell may be the answer not only to why there is a variety of responses to radiation but to why some people age faster than others.

In an effort to delve further into this aspect of radiation and aging, University of California researchers at Davis have been working with beagle dogs since 1954.

In 1954 they took a control group of dogs that would not be submitted to radiation and divided them in half. One half were given to people in the community to raise as pets and the other half were kept in the laboratory. Dogs given to private citizens lived an average of only 4.5 years. Dogs kept in the laboratory lived an average of 12.2 years.

In an irradiated group, dogs given a single large dose of 300 rads lived an average of 9.2 years and those exposed to 100 rads lived an average of 10.5 years. Tumors in the irradiated group were more prevalent than in the control group, but degenerative diseases such as kidney and hormone problems were more evident in the control group.

Yet, even the dogs receiving the highest doses of radiation were able to have litters, causing the researchers to question the difference in effects of radiation between species. Rodent ovaries are very susceptible to radiation and irradiated mice mothers produce defective offspring. Pregnant women who receive radiation have been found to produce children with a greater susceptibility to cancer. Such observations reinforce the idea that the cells of certain species may be more susceptible to attack by radiation and other mutagens and therefore may age faster. This may also explain the difference in life-spans between species.

But, if radiation causes aging by mutation, then other mutation-causing substances should also age the cell and its owner. Yet, when nitrogen mustard, a powerful mutagenic agent, was administered to animals in sublethal doses, no effect on aging and life-span was found, even when the agent was administered as often as three times a week for over two-thirds of the normal life-span of the animals.

But a closer look did not disprove the mutagenic theory of aging but reinforced it. Nitrogen mustard is a mutagenic substance, but it works on bone marrow and intestinal cells, both of which undergo rapid division. Remember that cells that undergo rapid division are able to throw off damaged mutant cells.

The nondivision of cells affects motherhood. We know that in both mice and men, the offspring of relatively old mothers have more defects and a shorter life-span than the offspring of young mothers. Even if the age of the father has any effect on this, researchers believe it is very small. Fathers have sperm cells, which continually divide and therefore can throw off mutations. Mothers have egg cells, which stay in the ovary and do not divide. The longer the nondividing egg stays in the ovary, the greater its possibility of accumulating mutations.

Drinking a cup of coffee or eating a piece of bologna, strange as it may seem, may contribute to your aging. Caffeine and the bologna (which has a meat preservative—sodium nitrate) may damage chromosomes. The body normally repairs some chromosome damage, but aging occurs when the balance of deterioration tips too far. Among other chemical mutagens in the environment capable of affecting human DNA are drugs, pesticides, food additives, known cancer-producing compounds, crude extracts of water, and atmospheric pollution.

Another widely acknowledged theory of aging is "cross-linking." At the beginning of World War II a thirty-four-year-old biochemist, Dr. Johan Bjorksten of Madison, Wis-

consin, published a paper stating that large molecules within
the cell, such as DNA, form bonds with other molecules and
become immobilized. What causes the molecules to hook together and become inseparable is still unknown. What is
known is that once they are hooked together, they can no
longer function adequately.

Cross-linking occurs outside the cell, particularly in collagen, one of the four major components of connective tissue.
Such cross-linking makes the collagen less elastic and so you
develop the characteristic joint and muscle stiffness of old age.

The body contains many agents, such as copper and
enzymes, believed to be capable of causing such cross-linking
Some cross-linking is believed to occur when more food is
ingested than can be immediately utilized. Other cross-linkers
are believed to be radiation, tobacco, smoke, and smog.

Some inert material from aged human hearts—a pigment—
has been purported to be the result of cross-linked molecules.
Also, mutagenic substances that produce cross-linking report-
edly shorten the average life-span much more than mutagenic
substances lacking the cross-linking agents.

However, the cross-linking theory of aging has lost
ground. While certainly there is cross-linking of molecules,
and consequently stiffness in tendons, cartilage, and skin, it
is apparently the *result* of the aging process and not the cause.
Cross-linking inside the cell, where the machinery of life
really is, has never been proven. It is just an outside phenomena.

Aging may be caused by a "clinker" in the cell. These
clinkers are evidently "ashes" from the fires of cell processes.
They can actually be seen as brown pigment and may occupy
as much as 30 percent of a cell's volume.

The idea is that clinkers build up and disrupt or choke
off the life of the cells. There is some evidence to link clinkers
with lysosomes—cavities within the cells that contain enzymes
capable of digesting parts of the cell. Lysosomes are nick-
named "suicide sacs" because in a number of conditions such
as starvation and deprivation of hormones, walls of the suicide
sacs break down and the lysosomes digest the surrounding

cellular material. When the material has been digested, there remains a complex of fat and proteins indistinguishable from the pigment clinkers. Lysosomes have also been linked to arthritis—acute inflammation of the joints and chronic inflammation of the joints, with cartilage erosion. A number of agents that explode lysosomes, such as the antibiotic streptomycin S and too much vitamin A, provoke inflammation and induce experimental arthritis.

Whether the brown pigment in cells is due to lysosomes or some other factor, there is no doubt that there is more of it in "old" cells than in "young" cells, but whether that pigment actually harms the cell is yet to be proven.

Immunity is also involved in aging. Studies show that 90 percent of the deaths in the United States each year result principally from the progressive loss of resistance to disease with advancing age.

The lack of resistance to disease in older people is well known, but it may be that not only does our immune mechanism not protect us in later years, but that it works against us. That is, mutations in cells may cause the cells to stimulate an unwarranted defensive reaction in the body. We become "allergic" to ourselves and our bodies eventually age and destroy themselves. Arthritis is believed to be such an immunologic disease and it does occur with greater frequency in old age. However, there are a number of elderly who never acquire any apparent immunologic disease. Nevertheless, in tests on mice, twenty-two animals were given a drug, Imuran, which suppresses immune reactions, and twenty-five were not. Those given Imuran lived 10 percent longer than those not given the drug, although all eventually succumbed to ordinary causes of mouse death.

Also, there are the everyday stresses of life that can cause wear and tear on the cells of the body. Dr. Hans Selye, an eminent Canadian researcher, maintains we all are born with a certain amount of "adaptation energy" that permits us to make adjustments to metabolic wounds caused by such stresses as disease, infection, accidents, exposure, worry, and malnutrition. Each stress situation draws upon our reserve of adaptation energy. Aging comes when the reserve begins to develop serious deficits.

Accordingly, there would be no distinction between alterations produced by age and those produced by disease, because very stressful episodes are fundamental components of the aging process. Every stress supposedly leaves an indelible scar, and the organism "pays for its survival after a stressful situation by becoming a little older." This is called the "watchspring theory." The human body supposedly is wound up and set for a certain length of time. When the watch spring winds down, we die.

Almost daily now, there are reports from around the world that add pieces to the puzzle of aging. We have from the University of Southern California, for instance, an "inhibitor" that supposedly "turns off" the cell's production of proteins and causes it to age. This inhibitor is programmed into the cell's code of life and occurs at a time when the cell is scheduled to age and die. No one has yet found the inhibitor but many are looking for it.

An oily substance that's chemically akin to motor oil may keep arteries young and flexible. This "oil" puts most of the spring in elastin, which makes connective tissue elastic. A loss of elasticity in elastin would go far to explain the development of hardening of the arteries.

Dr. Lawrence B. Sandberg of the University of Utah and his colleagues believe something causes the oily elastin molecule to flip-flop so that it rejects water instead of favoring it. The switch would cause elastin to lose its stretchability and make the artery hard. Dr. Sandberg and his group believe when they fully understand what happens to this oily substance, they can prevent its deterioration and therefore prevent deterioration of the arteries.

All these theories and observations have logic and experimental support as well as "holes." The exact cause of aging is yet to be proven, although, ironically, the answer to why we age may come not from the gerontology laboratory but from the cancer laboratory. Cancer and aging are just two sides of the coin. With cancer, the control mechanism goes awry and there is unregulated growth and cell division. With aging, the control mechanism goes awry and the cell dies.

If scientists find the answer to one, they will have the answer to both.

Although gerontologists and oncologists believe they are closing in on the answers in their respective fields, it may not be necessary for either to discover the exact mechanisms of why we age or why we get cancer. As with other disease, it may be possible to control the symptoms with chemicals and environmental manipulation without ever isolating the exact causes. With cancer, which is not fully understood, some forms can now be cured with surgery, chemicals, and radiation if diagnosed early. Some forms of aging can also be cured if diagnosed early.

Summing it up, there are two main approaches to the control of aging. One is to protect the DNA of the cell from attack by radiation, cross-linking, or other mutagens. The other is to slow down the preset program or to at least let an individual live out his or her full time.

As you will read in the following chapters, progress has already been made in both approaches and exciting information is rapidly being acquired.

Chapter 4

You Are as Young as Your Hormones

WHEN GOD TOOK A RIB from Adam's side to make a woman, He must have added an extra ingredient because the female of the species is biologically stronger and longer lasting than the male.

Although more human males are conceived, their attrition rate in the womb is higher—about 160 aborted or stillbirth males for every 100 females. In twin pregnancies, when male and female compete for survival, the female wins.

The life expectancy of the American woman has increased by 12½ years in the last three decades, while the life-span of the American male has lengthened only eight years. Females in the United States are rapidly outpopulating the males. In 1940 there were 500,000 more women than men in this country. In 1970, 5,401,869. The number of women in excess of men has increased more than five times in a period in which the population has not quite doubled.

What is that extra ingredient in women that makes them live longer? For a number of scientists, the answer is simple —the female hormone, estrogen. Still other scientists believe it is not estrogen that is beneficial, but the male hormone, testosterone, which is detrimental. All scientists, however, agree that hormones are intimately involved with how long and how well we live. They are the major factors, perhaps the hands of the biological time clock that determine how fast we age and why some people age faster than others.

Since Professor Arnold Berthold of Germany transplanted sex glands to the chests of two desexed roosters in 1848 and the capons began again to chase the chicks around the coop, mankind has looked upon hormones as potential elixirs of youth. According to current research, they may well be!

What are hormones? The word "hormone" for the substance secreted by the endocrine glands is derived from the Greek word "hormao," meaning "I arouse to activity."

The largest of the hormone secreters, the pancreas, has an average weight of less than three ounces. The smallest, the mysterious pineal, is about the size of a grape seed. All the others together—the thyroid, the four parathyroids, the twin adrenals, the pituitary, the thymus, and the paired ovaries of women or testes of men—weigh between four and seven ounces.

Yet, as tiny as they are, these mighty glands oversee our very lives and behavior. They control the process by which we digest our food and turn it into blood, bone, muscles, and brain. They make us tall or short, fat or thin. They regulate our heartbeat and affect the workings of our liver and kidneys. They set the time when a girl becomes a woman and a boy a man. They determine fertility, sexual behavior, and personality.

When we are attacked by a foe—either human or germ—they mobilize our defenses.

Of all the endocrines, the sex glands are the ones most associated in the public mind with aging. Men worry about them because they fear a drop in potency as the years go by; women, because they associate the cessation of the menses with a loss of sexual desirability. (See Chapter 9.)

When a French professor at the Sorbonne, Charles Brown-Sequard, in 1869 injected extract of dog testicle into himself and claimed it made him potent and vigorous, he was a hundred years ahead of his time. His experiments were judged failures by the medical men of the era and set the infant science of endocrinology back for years.

We know today that the male hormone, testosterone, does indeed affect potency. However, the male hormone may be a liability as well as a joy. Acne and baldness are dependent upon male hormones.

Three possible explanations are possible for the difference in survival rate between men and women—stress, sex chromosomes, and sex hormones.

Research has found that bigger stresses are not applied to males. Males can't withstand many of the stresses endured by females. A higher percentage of male heavy smokers suffer from cancer than do female heavy smokers. Likewise, the decrease in life-span for the obese is greater for men than for women.

The second explanation, the sex chromosome, is intimately tied with the sex hormone theory. A chromosome is a unit of a cell that carries genetic information. In mammals, a female has two X chromosomes, while a male has only one X and a much smaller Y chromosome.

Some people believe that the second X protects women. However, it may be the small Y chromosome that is detrimental to the male. In both the human species and in lower forms of life, there are certain "supermales" who have two Y chromosomes instead of an X and a Y. A number of these supermales have been found in prison; scientists theorize the double Y constitutes an innate aggressiveness and intimate its existence may foretell future inmates.

YY chromosome male animals have shorter life expectancies than normal XY males, a confirmation for science that genetic and hormonal factors may be involved in male life expectancy.

As for the third explanation for differences in survival rates, the sex hormone, castrated males live significantly longer than normal males, especially if the castration takes place before puberty, whether they are tomcats or humans.

In contrast to former centuries when castration was performed on singers in churches and opera houses, as well as on personnel in harems and imperial palaces, the operation is now done chiefly in cases of prostatic cancer (which is linked to male sex hormones; see Chapter 9) and on mentally retarded or psychotic males.

In a long-term study of institutionalized mentally retarded males, 735 intact and 297 eunuchs, each eunuch was matched closely with one or more intact males for such characteristics as year of birth and length of hospitalization. Because they are mentally retarded, the subjects had only a vague idea of the effects of castration, which reduced any possible adverse psychological effects of the operation.

Thus far the average life-span for the intact males is 55.7 and 69.3 years for eunuchs. The younger the males are castrated, the longer they live. However, for most males, obviously, when it comes to a choice between virility and a longer life, they'd choose virility.

The study also indicated that the castrated are less susceptible to infections. This is believed to be due to the antibody-lowering effect of testosterone reported by some researchers. Antibodies are the body's own disease fighters.

The evidence for more virile men dying younger seems to be building. Statistics show that ambitious, aggressive men are more prone to heart disease than others. Recent studies under grants from the National Institutes of Health show that the higher the level of testosterone, the more aggressive the man.

However, it may not be testosterone that causes the divergence in survival between men and women, but the hormone estrogen. In her entire lifetime, a woman produces barely two tablespoonfuls of the female hormones, estrogen and progesterone, yet the survival of the human race depends upon the release and perfect synchronization of microscopic amounts of these substances.

In most creatures the reproductive cycle and life itself are closely intertwined. When one ends, so does the other. Yet, the twentieth-century American woman lives almost as many years after menopause as before.

Still for a large percentage of women, menopause is a traumatic experience. It usually occurs just as their children are grown and leaving home, and their husbands are at the apex of their careers. Many women feel that with their reproduction function finished, they are old and useless.

The physical symptoms of menopause are well known,

passed from mother to daughter, from girl friend to girl friend through the generations. The main manifestations are hot flashes, nervousness, irritability, and insomnia. There may also be accompanying dizziness, headache, joint and muscle pain, numbness, and severe depression. The vagina, urethra (the tube that carries the urine), and breast tissue may atrophy. The skin loses moisture and supporting fat, and it begins to wrinkle.

A significant number of women experience no uncomfortable symptoms. Others (and consequently their families) suffer severe problems.

Menopause actually consists of two stages. The first is a change in the menstrual pattern, and the second the end of ovulation itself. In the first stage the ovaries gradually slow down their production of both estrogen and progesterone. The menstrual flow becomes irregular and more widely spaced. In some cases it stops abruptly. The egg follicles form but do not reach maturity.

During her fertile period a woman's pituitary gland and her ovaries work in concert to maintain a delicate balance. As the ovaries begin to slow down, the pituitary gets excited and produces more ovary-stimulating hormones, but to no avail. The intricate glandular balance becomes upset and the acute symptoms occur. When a new adjustment is made, the acute symptoms disappear.

However, after hot flashes and other acute symptoms disappear, new problems appear. Many statistical, clinical, and experimental studies reveal that estrogen protects women against heart disease. When young women have their ovaries removed surgically, their heart attack rate equals men's, which is three times greater than that of premenopausal women. How estrogen protects women is not clear, although it is believed to have a cholesterol-lowering effect.

But estrogen has not been therapeutic in treating or preventing heart disease. In fact, the Coronary Drug Project, sponsored by the National Heart and Lung Institute, dropped the use of the hormone from the study because of the high number of nonfatal heart attacks and blood clots in the lung associated with it.

The Veterans Administration cooperative study on cancer of the prostate also showed higher mortality from coronary heart disease in the estrogen-treated males. Therefore, if the hormone does protect premenopausal women, it is not yet in a form that can transfer this protection to men.

Estrogen also protects the bone of women. The bones of postmenopausal women begin to become porous, brittle, and susceptible to collapse and fracture when the level of this hormone falls. The lack of estrogen is believed to cause a negative balance of protein, calcium, and other bone-nourishing minerals. Such women literally "shrink" as their spinal columns become shorter and they develop "dowager's hump," a stooped posture characteristic of many older women. Men, on the other hand, continue to secrete testosterone in sufficient amounts until much later in life when their bones also may become fragile.

Since 1940 physicians have found that by administering estrogen to postmenopausal women, they could ease or completely alleviate the acute symptoms of menopause, the hot flashes, irritability, and the other manifestations.

At first the doctors gave estrogen only to the estrogen-deficient women for a very short period of time. One physician, Dr. Robert A. Wilson, began prescribing estrogen for postmenopausal women indefinitely.

He maintained that when you find a woman of fifty looking like thirty, or a woman of sixty looking and acting like forty, chances are that she is one of the lucky ones who have benefited from the new techniques of menopausal prevention. The outward signs of this age-defying youthfulness are straight-backed posture, supple breast contours, taut, smooth skin on face and neck, firm muscle tone, and that particular vigor and grace typical of a healthy female. At fifty, such women still look attractive in tennis shorts or sleeveless dresses.

Should you take estrogen? Most physicians will not prescribe supplemental estrogen unless a woman shows definite signs of estrogen deficiency. A number of women never do because their bodies continue to produce some estrogen or an estrogenlike hormone.

Since the ovary produces both estrogen and progesterone in premenopausal women, a few physicians give both hormones to postmenopausal women.

Estrogen and progesterone are the components of the birth control pill. One doctor believes that hormone-deficient postmenopausal women should continue to take both estrogen and progesterone, but on a slightly different schedule. Instead of taking the combination pill for twenty days and then stopping for ten, as premenopausal women do for birth control, he prescribes taking estrogen for twenty days and then progesterone for ten days. Women on this routine continue to menstruate indefinitely.

Progesterone causes the endometrial lining of the uterus to break down each month. This action is the basis for the fear that some physicians hold about giving progesterone to postmenopausal women. They are afraid of inducing endometrial cancer. They are also afraid of inducing breast cancer with the estrogen in the pill. Breast cancer, the biggest cancer killer of women, occurs most frequently in postmenopausal women.

In experiments with a more than one thousand postmenopausal women on the combination pill for over ten years, there have been no incidents of endometrial cancer and only two cases of breast cancer. In that period, according to current statistics, there should have been fifty cases of breast cancer.

An estrogen side effect that has physicians worried is its apparent ability to cause blood clots in susceptible women. The incidence, although small, has been frequent enough to cause the Federal Food and Drug Administration to require such a warning on the contraceptive pill's container.

Apparently, such blood clotting has not been a problem in postmenopausal women. The explanation is that a different type of estrogen is used and it is given in much smaller doses than in the birth control pill.

Can hormones really control the aging process? One way to find out is to take an ovary from a young woman and transplant it into an older woman. If the ovary remains young, if it has not been taken over by the body's machinery, there is no central hormonal control. If it ages rapidly, there must exist some overall control.

Among patients who have undergone a transplant of ovaries, some who had never ovulated began ovulating with the transplant. An Italian physician took an ovary from a thirty-year-old woman and transplanted it into a twenty-four-year-old woman. The woman whose own ovaries had been removed began to have twenty-eight-day menstrual cycles, with appropriate temperature variation. It is possible that in this example the ovary was responding to the stimulus of a master gland, the pituitary. Further research will determine whether the pituitary of an older woman will stimulate a youthful, transplanted ovary.

Birth control researchers are working along these lines. They are seeking to isolate a chemical from the master hormone control center, the hypothalamus. The chemicals, hypothalamic leutinizing hormone releasing factors (LRF), act on the pituitary gland which in turn secretes hormones to ripen and release the egg from the ovary. The ovary, in turn, secretes a hormone that, in sort of a feedback, influences the release of LRF.

What the drug researchers are trying to do is to develop an imitation LRF pill that will confuse the pituitary or ovary hormones and interfere with the reproductive cycle. The new pills will be more specific, affecting just reproduction and not the other body systems as the estrogen-progesterone pills now do. But once isolated, the LRF can be used to maintain the proper levels of hormones as well as to block them. This could keep the hormones in balance as we age.

Men undergo a sort of menopause—a male climacteric. Symptoms appear between fifty and sixty years in some men, including easy fatigue, difficulty in concentrating, failing memory, and restlessness, with sleeplessness and heightened irritability or irascibility. Some men also experience weight loss, weakness, muscular aches and pains, constipation, dizziness, anginal pain, and a decrease in the force of the urinary stream. Impotency is among the least common complaints.

Supplementary male hormone sometimes alleviates these "menopause" symptoms. However, not for long, because there is a wearing-off effect. The few doses of testosterone do not work to the same degree as does estrogen for the female symptoms.

Women are luckier. Although estrogen and progesterone replacement will not keep women young forever, the hormones do retard the aging process, especially in those critical years. (We have seen that women age twenty-three years in ten calendar years between forty and fifty years—the time when estrogen makes its dramatic drop.)

But sex hormones, of course, are not the whole answer to the aging problem. Lack of another hormone, thyroxine, also causes symptoms that very much resemble old age. The skin becomes dry and thick, the hair coarse, and the face puffy. The thyroid-deficient victim becomes slow, sluggish, and fat.

Stimulated by the pituitary to produce its own hormone, the thyroid can speed up the rate of metabolism, the rate at which the body uses its food materials, and then keep it at the proper level so that the body's use of food proceeds at an efficient rate. The slowdown of the thyroid's production may be one reason why people are always saying: "I don't eat any more than I did when I was younger, but I really put on weight now."

Not enough thyroid can affect any of the body's systems. It many cause arthritis-like symptoms, deafness, nearsightedness, and even mental retardation or mental illness. It can clog the arteries with cholesterol and lead to heart ailments.

Although such symptoms occur in old age, the major decrease in thyroid function actually occurs around puberty. The slowdown of this gland in later years is relatively small.

However, when supplementary thyroid hormones are given to older persons, they seem to have little effect. This may be due to the presence of an "inhibitor" released by the pituitary gland, which would come into play at puberty and gradually shut off the effectiveness of the thyroid hormone.

If this pituitary inhibitor could be found, and the theory proves correct, it may be counteracted and the signs of old age associated with hypothyroidism may be eliminated.

A thyroid hormone, thyrocalcitonin, is believed to transfer calcuim from the blood to the bone, the opposite function of parathyroids, which control the removal of calcium from the bone into the blood. With infusions of calcium we can stimulate calcitonin and suppress the parathyroids, thereby benefiting patients suffering from osteoporosis—bone fragility. Osteoporosis is frequently involved in backaches in people over fifty years of age.

Until very recently scientists believed that the pituitary, which is between the top of the mouth and the base of the brain, was the "master gland" because it releases substances that stimulate or depress most of the other endocrine glands. Now we know that the pituitary merely takes orders from the hypothalamus, a control center at the base of the brain and perhaps the real mastermind of aging.

It is the hypothalamus that produces chemicals that stimulate or prevent the release of hormones from the pituitary gland. In turn, the hormones released by the pituitary gland stimulate the target glands, such as the thyroid or the adrenal, which in turn release their own hormones to affect various body functions.

But then an American physiologist won a Nobel Prize for, in effect, telling hormone researchers there was more to it than that. Dr. Earl Sutherland isolated a substance, cyclic adenosine 3′5′ monophosphate, called Cyclic AMP for short, which occurs in trace amounts in every human cell. Hormones drop their messages at a cell's door, cyclic AMP picks up the message and carries it inside to do its work. Dr. Sutherland calls his discovery "the second messenger."

There is so much research now going on with cyclic AMP

that no one can keep up with it, but Sutherland's discovery
has great potential against cancer. In more than half a dozen
laboratories, cyclic AMP can kill off cancer cells in a dish
or return them to normal.

Cyclic AMP studies around the world provide valuable
information on mental illness and heart, stomach, parathyroid,
adrenal, and sex gland disorders, as well as on how the body
ages.

But cyclic AMP is not the only missing link recently discovered in the hormone chain reaction. There are prostaglandins, intriguing substances that will not only be used to
treat the ills afflicting the aged, but possibly even to prevent
or retard aging itself.

Prostaglandins took their name from their discovery, in
the early 1930s, in the prostate glands of sheep. Later, these
substances were also found in lesser amounts in the uterus,
lungs, thymus, pancreas, and kidney tissue. Prostaglandins
may exist in almost all—if not all—tissues.

But not until 1959 did anything come of these curious
chemicals, when Dr. Sune Bergstrom and other scientists in
Sweden isolated two prostaglandins in pure crystalline form.
Furthermore, when they administered them to humans it increased the heart rate and caused a slight drop in arterial blood
pressure. In the early 1970s prostaglandins helped terminate
pregnancies successfully by their infusion into the patients'
veins.

There are now more than fourteen known prostaglandins,
and others are being sought. All resemble each other in structure but have greatly different effects. Various prostaglandins
can induce childbirth and abortion, correct male sterility and
control female fertility, lower blood pressure, alleviate asthma,
stop the secretion of stomach acid in ulcer victims, open
clogged nasal passages, and soothe such inflammatory ills as
arthritis.

Prostaglandins have great medicinal potential for a wide
range of ills—from arthritis to high blood pressure and, by
controlling such diseases, they will greatly affect how we

age. What is not certain is just how they fit into the hormone cycle.

Prostaglandins may either stimulate the production and accumulation of cyclic AMP or block its formation altogether. The action depends on the tissue and the cells. In other words, scientists now believe the hormone system works like this: Picture a baseball game. The pituitary-pitcher throws the ball to the batter, a target endocrine, such as the thyroid gland. The batter-endocrine then hits the ball to the target organ, or first base. The first baseman is cyclic AMP, ready to receive the ball. However, the first-base coach, prostaglandin, either tells the first baseman, cyclic AMP, to catch the ball or let it go by.

How fast we age may depend on how well these hormone baseball players work together.

Probably the most mysterious of the endocrines and one which may play a large part in aging is the pineal. It is a small bulge of brain deep between the two hemispheres. It is glandular in appearance in the young, and hard and stony in older people. It has long been thought to be a leftover, as has the appendix, from a more primitive form of life because in some animals it is located between the eyes and has photoreceptive cells. It was considered a vestigal third eye.

The pineal may be the "arm" of a biological clock. For a long time we have known there are biological clocks within our bodies that keep time even in the absence of external stimuli, such as day-night changes in lighting. They regulate body functions and a whole new field of medicine is being built around this phenomenon. Whether there is a central clock or many clocks is not known, nor is it known how these timers communicate regulating information to distant parts of the body.

The most striking circadian (about a day) rhythm in the body occurs in the serotonin content of the rat pineal gland. The level of serotonin—an important nerve hormone—varies from a low at midnight to peak levels three times higher at noon. The cycle repeats itself regularly every twenty-four hours.

Three serotonin rhythms are timed by a true biological clock, since they continue to function in rats kept in constant darkness, as well as in blinded animals. When the day-night cycle is reversed for one week, the pineal serotonin rhythm also reverses, so that the lowest level occurs at noon, and the highest at midnight. When the nerve connections from the central nervous system to the pineal gland are cut, the pineal rhythm ceases and the level of serotonin remains halfway between the usual noon peak and the midnight low.

Does the pineal determine the timers of our aging? Or is it merely a "relay station" for the real but as yet undiscovered central clock? Work on the pineal is still relatively in the early stages.

A better understood gland but one which also seems to affect aging is the adrenal, so named because it lies on top of the kidneys (ad-renal). The two adrenals are responsible for among other things the regulation of the amounts of salt and potassium present in the blood stream. Without these chemicals the nervous system and the cells of the body die. The adrenals also produce several hormones similar to those produced by the sex glands. In addition, the adrenals secrete substances that prepare the body to "fight or flee." However, too much adrenalin may possibly "stress" the body and perhaps cause it to "age."

The largest of the hormone secreters, the pancreas, affects the amount of sugar in the blood and produces juices to aid digestion. Among the problems of old age is the inability to digest proteins and to tolerate sugar. But we still don't know what causes the pancreas to slow down as we age.

Perhaps the most exciting work with hormones and aging today concerns the thymus gland. Located at the upper part of the chest, it lies over the trachea under the first of several ribs. Its exact function is still unknown. It appears to be active in childhood and gradually regresses and becomes smaller as growth reaches its limit. Many believe that aging begins when growth reaches its limit, and therefore it is quite possible that the thymus is the gland that triggers aging.

Until 1961 nothing at all was known about the gland.

Then, Dr. Jacques F. A. P. Miller of the Chester Beatty Institute, England, removed the thymus from newborn mice. For several weeks after the operation, the baby mice seemed to thrive. But after that, they fell ill and ultimately died of a disease marked by rapid weight loss and diarrhea.

There is also Sir F. MacFarlane Burnet's immune theory of aging; the English Nobel Prize winner believes that the body becomes "allergic" to itself and self-destructs and that there are three factors:

• Aging in any species is genetically programmed as a result of evolutionary processes.

• The program is mediated essentially by a built-in metabolic clock.

• Organs, or physiological systems, will differ widely in the time needed to use up their quota of cells. Many systems never approach their limits, but that system, vital to life, which first uses up its quota will be the chief secondary mediator of aging.

Everything points to the thymus-dependent (TD) immune system as the key system whose exhaustion is responsible for aging in mammals and probably other vertebrates. Remember that the thymus shrivels early in childhood. It is true that if the most essential function of the thymus system is to deal with abnormal cells, then the system may control cancer and autoimmune diseases such as arthritis.

This theory seems reinforced in that rats with their thymus removed are highly susceptible to spontaneous cancer.

Among other symptoms found in thymectomized rodents were gray hair, thin translucent skin, and loss of body fat. When autopsied, the rodents had many different abnormalities, including heart disease, widespread amyloid deposits, severe kidney disease, and destruction of the liver and pancreas. There were widespread tumors.

Apparently, the removal of the thymus may either allow the growth of dormant malignant cells or allow bacterial or viral infections to set off the tumor process.

As pointed out before, the reason humans die of so-called

"old age" is usually because they are no longer immune to diseases. Although the cause of death may be listed as "cancer" or "heart disease" when autopsied, an older person may have had as many as twenty-five different diseases present in the body, a situation similar to the one found in thymectomized mice.

The destruction of the thymus may account for the destruction of the body known as "aging."

If so, would it be possible to take a piece of our thymus when we are young, freeze it, and give it back to us when we are older?

This is just what was suggested by eminent immunologists at a science writers' conference in 1971. And indeed, in 1972, two successful thymus transplants were performed in infants to give them missing immunity.

In immunology, we may discover a giant step toward the control of aging.

There are actually two types of immunologic protection in the body. One is the "T" cell from the thymus, which protects against viral and some bacterial infections. The other is the "B" cell derived from bone marrow, which protects against bacterial infections. A large percentage of the "B" cells are manufactured in the spleen.

Certain diseases such as arthritis may be related to the overproduction of "B" cells. Such diseases occur more frequently in old age. The theory is that the "B" cells overdo their intended protection against invading bacteria and cause inflammation and damage as the years go by.

In the meantime the thymus becomes less effective as we age and we lose our protection against viral disease. In fact, it is possible that aging symptoms are caused by long dormant viruses that come to life as our defenses wane. This fits right into the observation that today's victims of parkinsonism were yesterday's victims of severe influenza infections.

It would also explain why cancer is more prevalent in older age groups. Many cancers are thought to be due to viruses.

Another piece in the puzzle fits if the immunologists are correct. They say the "T" cells have the power to turn off the production of "B" cells, thus preventing destruction of tissue by an overabundance of the bacteria fighters. On the other hand, the "B" cells have the power to turn off the "T" cells. As we age, we lose "T" cells, which in turn allow the overproduction of "B" cells, but these "B" cells in turn allow the killing off of more "T" cells.

With a thymus transplant in later years, we would then, if the theory is correct, have sufficient "T" cells to fight off viruses and to keep a rein on "B" cells to prevent arthritis and other autoimmune diseases.

Another important step in the understanding of aging was the synthesis of the pituitary's human growth hormone, HGH, in 1971. The synthetic hormone has about 10 percent of the growth-producing properties of the natural one.

Human growth hormone was first isolated in 1956. It has a profound effect on many body functions, including the metabolism of sugar, fats, and proteins. In the male the growth hormone promotes the activity of the male hormone, androgen. In the female, sex hormones function more effectively with HGH. Growth hormone also increases the production of disease-fighting antibodies.

An excess of natural growth hormone can cause children (before puberty) to grow into giants. After puberty, an excess affects only the head and limbs. A lack of the hormone causes dwarfism.

Growth hormone may be associated with cancer growth. Surgeons have removed pituitaries from women with breast cancer leading to some remissions. In rats, whose growth hormone producing pituitaries have been removed, injection of cancer-inducing substances and viruses seem to have no effect. But if the animals are then given growth hormone, cancer develops even though the hormone by itself does not initiate cancerous growth.

The synthesis of growth hormone has had a profound effect on aging research. Until it was made in the laboratory there was not enough of it to experiment with. We do know that growth hormone can affect the nitrogen, fat and water components of the body—even in old animals. Seriously ill or very aged people may go into negative nitrogen balance and lose protein. Such people become weak and emaciated. When growth hormone is administered, this condition improves.

Growth hormone has already been very good therapy for osteoporosis in dogs, and it may yet help humans suffering from the bone problem.

Human growth hormone may be the same as the so-called juvenile hormone in lower forms of life. If so, we may all be able to grow new fingers, toes, and limbs if we need them.

Creatures like the cockroach have the ability to regenerate missing limbs when young. However, once the cockroach grows old, it loses this ability.

In experiments at the University of Virginia, tiny holes were bored in the backs of young and old cockroaches, which were then fused so that their body fluids mixed. The legs of the old cockroaches were then amputated and they promptly grew new ones. The juvenile hormone from the young cockroach enabled the old cockroaches to grow new legs.

If the juvenile hormone is the same as human growth hormone, could this regeneration be achieved in humans? Yes, according to researchers at the Syracuse Veterans Hospitals. They believe that with proper electrical stimulation of cellular activity, the specific hormone would be released to enable limb regeneration in humans.

The frog, like the human, does not grow new limbs. Yet, frogs regenerate limb cells. When they were electrically stimulated, the cells de-differentiated, that is, they changed back into cells capable of becoming something else, as if they were embryo cells.

If frog cells can de-differentiate, then presumably so can human cells. By affecting the proper hormone balance with electricity, human cells that once had the ability to regenerate long ago in evolution, may once again have it. Within twenty or thirty years, eminent researchers believe we will be able to grow new digits and limbs if we need them. Right now, of course, electrical stimulation is being used successfully to speed the healing of bones in patients with fractures.

Summing up, there is more evidence concerning the links

between hormones and aging than perhaps any other physiological process in the human body. Hormones are already being used to prevent some symptoms of aging. If the hormones can be kept in harmony indefinitely, our song of life may indeed be greatly extended.

Chapter 5

Mind Over Matter

PERHAPS THE MOST FEARED aspect of aging is the loss of mental prowess.

We do lose brain cells. After the age of thirty, we lose several thousand cerebral cells each day; the brain decreases in bulk, so that by age seventy-five it is slightly over 50 percent of its original weight. For many people intellectual functions peak and fade early; on average, number memory begins to decline after age twenty-five, design memory after age thirty, inductive reasoning after twenty, and tonal memory after forty-five.

Yet, some people never seem to lose their intellectual abilities, even in extreme old age. George Bernard Shaw, for instance, was still writing creatively at ninety-four years; Picasso was busy painting on his ninetieth birthday; Bernard Baruch was still advising presidents just before he died at ninety-five years; Charles G. Abbot, one of America's foremost astrophysicists, celebrated his one hundredth birthday by filing for a patent on a radically new zero-pollution solar engine.

Our memories usually give us the first clue that our minds are not as sharp as they once were. But David Roth, the memory expert, could still recite Thomas Gray's 128-line "Elegy Written in a Country Churchyard," cite the day of the week for any date from 1752 to 3000, and repeat the telephone numbers of any of the six hundred members in his chapter of the Rotary Club on his ninety-seventh birthday.

If brain researchers are correct in that we lose brain cells in adulthood each day, we are all going to become senile if we live long enough. Anyone who maintains good mental faculties into very old age does so because, for a variety of reasons, he doesn't lose brain cells as fast as others.

Is there anything we can do to prevent the intellectual decline associated with loss of brain cells during aging? There is. Furthermore, as knowledge increases about how the brain ages, compounds will be developed to keep the mind functioning at maximum capacity. In fact, there are already memory medications in work as you will read later in the chapter.

The central control of aging in the whole body is believed to be located in the brain. In the chapter on hormones, we saw that the hypothalamus at the base of the brain is the real master gland. It controls the functioning of the endocrine glands, which in turn regulate the functioning of the body. Furthermore, the brain may determine the actual rate of aging. Why? Because those born with damaged brain cells—mongoloids and certain other categories of retardates—age more rapidly than anyone else. The mentally retarded die at an average age of thirty-eight years compared with sixty-two years for psychotics and sixty-eight to seventy years for the population at large. Mongoloids have eighteen times the incidence of leukemia and twenty-six times the incidence of cancer of the population at large. They also go bald in childhood and develop wrinkled skin at a very early age. Mongoloids and a number of other categories of retarded are born with broken chromosomes. The rest of us are believed to acquire broken chromosomes during a process we call aging.

The most spectacular of premature aging associated with mental retardation occurs in victims of progeria, an accelerated old age. A Brazilian boy, who died of the disease recently, began suffering from the symptoms at five months. He succumbed to a heart attack at the age of twelve, and when he was buried, he looked like a wizened old man of ninety.

Some of us who are born with a complete set of brain cells go about hastening their destruction. The loss of brain cells can be related directly to life-style. Those who are heavy smokers, drinkers, and drug addicts lose brain cells at an accelerated rate, as do those who take sleeping pills, don't eat properly, or overeat. Those who are depressed or who can't sleep also hasten the depletion of cells. And we may have practically a whole generation with premature loss of brain cells; studies done in Texas have shown that repeatedly smoking marijuana causes premature aging of the brain.

If we are ever to control or prevent brain cell loss, we must first understand how and when brain damage occurs. The electroencephalograph (EEG) is one approved aid. It measures the electrical activity of the brain, which is recorded on a sort of graph as a wave pattern. In a study of three hundred healthy individuals EEG patterns changed markedly during childhood and into adolescence and then remained somewhat stable until the age of forty. At forty the EEG tracings began to resemble those of sixty-five- to seventy-five-year-olds.

The EEG machine disclosed that while stimulus information reaches the brain in essentially the same amount of time in an eighty-six-year-old as in a seventeen-year-old, there is a lag in the brain's computer processing of the information. This delay correlates with the longer reaction time commonly seen in the elderly. However, the mature adult's larger "computer information bank" allows him to compensate for the slowness in computation and therefore to remain competitive with younger, quicker brains.

Although it hasn't been explained yet, the electrical amplitude from the right half of the brain is greater than from the left in normal individuals. Right-handedness or left-handedness has nothing to do with it. This difference, however, is less marked in dull children, absent in mongoloids, and vanishes in normal adults after they drink three ounces of alcohol, which changes the state of consciousness.

Past the age of forty there is an increasing incidence of irregular electrical rhythm over the left temporal lobe of the brain, above and in front of the ear. This is the area that controls memory, speech, and cognition; 20 percent of the adults between the ages of forty and forty-nine show this electrical offbeat rhythm. Between fifty and fifty-nine, there is a slight increase in the number, but after the age of sixty, 36 percent of those tested had the abnormality. However, those who did not show the change in the EEG by the age of seventy did not develop it.

Chances are that if Picasso or George Bernard Shaw had submitted to an EEG, even up to their last years, they would not have shown that rhythmic abnormality.

Can you prevent this change in your own brain waves? If you are a man, it will be harder for you than if you are a woman, but it can be done. First of all, you have to prevent or minimize hardening of the arteries. Women's brains develop arteriosclerosis more slowly. Males have changes in the arteries of their brains beginning in the third decade, while females do not have changes until the fifth decade.

You have to keep your blood pressure controlled so it doesn't go too high or too low. The changes in the electrical activity over the left temporal region mentioned before are believed to be due to changes in the blood supply to this area. A correlation between these changes and a definite decline in verbal abilities has been shown.

Blood pressure has also been correlated with intellect. A slight or moderately high blood pressure apparently is good for the brain. As blood vessels age, they are not as efficient at sending blood to the head, but when the pressure is turned up a little, sufficient blood keeps the brain in good working order.

On the other hand, high blood pressure is a major factor in intellectual decline. In elderly volunteers studied over a ten-year period, those who had normal or a little above normal blood pressure showed no intellectual deficit during the decade. Those who had high blood pressure showed a significant loss of mental acuity through the years. A maintenance of mental sharpness can therefore be aided by keeping blood pressure within bounds. This is possible today with proper medical care and drugs already on the market.

Prevention and care of heart damage can also keep the

brain in good working order. A watch on the brain could signal heart trouble long before an individual suspects its presence. In a study of healthy individuals the blood flow through the brain was essentially the same whether they were twenty-five or seventy-two years old. But when the brain waves tended to be slower in frequency, it signaled heart problems and poorer blood flow.

This also occurred in commercial airline pilots who suffered heart attacks. Such pilots have the same kind of slowed mental responses often found in the elderly.

Brain wave readings of persons kept in an environment deprived of most of the input through the five senses for several days showed a tendency toward slower brain waves seen in older people. But the brain waves reverted to normal as soon as those in the experiment were allowed to return to more sensory input.

This all demonstrates that if the brain receives sufficient blood from the heart and sufficient stimuli, it can function well even in old age.

A good night's sleep keeps the brain in good working order. There are four basic stages of sleep, starting with the light sleep of Stage 1 and progressing down to the deep sleep of Stage 4. Stage 4 sleep has been known to diminish toward the vanishing point as early as the late thirties or by the early forties.

When we sleep, we have rapid eye movements (REMs). With the aid of the EEG and the patient's own recollections, these periods of rapid eye movements signify dreaming. Not only do we dream during REMs, our heart rate increases, our cholesterol level rises, our blood pressure may go up, and we may sweat.

The number of REMs we have between the ages of five and ninety does not appear to change. However, children sleep two to three hours before their first REM. Young adults take an average of seventy-nine minutes before their first REMs appear, and aged people, fifty-eight minutes.

Although not entirely understood, REMs are important to mental well-being in both young and old. On specific tests on elderly patients, those who awakened often during the night and who showed a decline in REM sleep did less well on psychological tests than older people who slept well.

Beyond adolescence, we do not sleep longer at age twenty to thirty than we do at seventy to eighty. Young adults, however, take less time falling asleep and do not awaken so much at night. Older people obtain an equivalent amount of sleep but they must do so by remaining in bed a longer time. On the average, older people awake so much during the night that they spend 17 percent of their time in bed wakeful. Young adults spend most of their time in bed asleep.

By the age of forty-five, the average adult awakens about three times during the night, but the awakenings are so brief, they will not be remembered. An average person past sixty-five awakens five or more times a night. What does all this prove?

That loss of cognitive power seems in some way related to an inability to maintain a restful sleep. Insomnia and disturbed sleep patterns are not found in all older people. Therefore, it may well be that poor sleep is abnormal, if somewhat common in old age. Furthermore, much insomnia and restless sleep may be due to psychological problems rather than physiologic ones. Many older people have nothing to do during the day. They catnap and have no set routine. Therefore, they may awaken at night because they had sufficient sleep during the day.

A more active day mentally and physically would go far to reduce the sleeping problems and consequently the cognitive problems of many elderly insomniacs and restless sleepers.

What else can be done to prevent loss of intellect? Thinking, of course, involves memory and permits intellectual development. Recent memory is the memory that we use to learn new things. It gives us the most trouble as we age. That is why older people who do not practice mentally often lose it and live in the past.

The information we store in our brains comes to us almost entirely through our senses. Sight, smell, hearing, touch, taste, and temperature perception are our special or exterior senses.

They bring us all we need to know of the world around us. But there are also our interior senses—hunger, thirst, fatigue, and pain perception. Another sense, that of equilibrium, or balance, tells us of our position in space right side up or upside down. Still another sense, which has no popular name, tells us of our activity (with the aid of tiny receptors inside our muscles and joints); most of us aren't even aware we have it, and yet we all use this muscular sense to determine whether something is heavy, light, soft, hard, or gaseous.

We also have a mysterious sense of distance or space. We don't usually exercise this sense, but we all have it. As we walk down a dark hallway, for example, we become aware without touching the wall that the hallway ends. This may be due to changes in reflected sounds from the walls. This faculty has been developed, particularly in blind people.

Our senses tell us, at first very subtly, that we are aging. In most of us, but intriguingly not in all of us, the ability of the senses to perceive the stimuli in our internal and external environment gradually declines, sometimes beginning at a surprisingly early age.

For instance, about 90 percent of what we perceive comes through our sense of sight, yet presbyopia, loss of the ability of the lens to accommodate for near and distant vision, begins around the age of twelve. At that time the lens has already lost some of its flexibility. Between sixteen and ninety years, recovery time from exposure to glare is doubled every thirteen years. The aged driver is easily blinded by the glare of onrushing headlights and has difficulty distinguishing far objects.

Color vision is also affected because yellowing of the lens filters out blue. There is an increased need for illumination as we age and a decreased ability to distinguish varying intensities of light, a decreased speed of perception of light stimuli, and a narrowing of the visual field so that we see less and less out of the corners of our eyes.

Eye specialists, though they may not be able to prevent certain changes, can correct vision deficits easily with lenses and maintain the sight stimuli to our brains.

Ironically, ear specialists can also correct deficits in hearing, with a hearing aid, yet people who will accept glasses without question refuse to recognize the need for a hearing aid. Gerontologists have found that loss of hearing is more detrimental to the mental well-being of an aging person than moderate loss of sight. The stress of not hearing well causes mental irritation and at times withdrawal.

Loss of hearing is not a normal part of aging because in less civilized, quieter societies, hearing is as keen at seventy-five years as it is at eighteen years. A famous study of Maaban tribesmen, who live in the quiet back country of Africa, proved this.

Aging pilots seem to have a greater loss of hearing in their left ears than in their right. The explanation? When pilots are promoted to full-captain rank, they move from the right side of the cockpit to the left side, where their left ear is closer to the noise and vibration of the engines.

The generation of rock-and-roll fans probably will become hard of hearing at a much earlier age than their parents.

The loss of hearing as we age in our noisy society is due to damage to the inner ear and nerve. Higher frequencies are the first to go and, eventually, certain sounds may become painful.

But if too much noise makes us deaf, lack of noise as we age can affect us mentally. Background noise is necessary for mental health. When an aging person misses these subtle sounds, he may not realize it but he will, as a result, feel a sense of loss, a feeling that the world is dead. Gerontologists recommend increasing, not decreasing, the background noise in retirement homes so as to keep the elderly in contact with the environment.

The conclusion? If you want to keep your hearing, and consequently your mind young, stay away from loud noises. If you are not hearing as well as you used to, seek the advice of a physician and if he recommends a hearing aid, accept it.

There is little doubt that wear and tear ages the senses. By the age of sixty years, for instance, most people have lost 50 percent of their taste buds and 40 percent of their ability to smell. This may explain why older people do not enjoy eating and drinking as much as the young.

Of course, there are compensations. You don't hurt as much physically. Studies show that the most striking drop in pain sensitivity occurs between forty and forty-nine years and again between fifty and fifty-nine years.

Since the input of the senses are received in the brain, the aging of the brain must also affect the senses as well as vice versa.

Some changes have actually seen seen in brain cells. These are the so-called age pigments, believed to be either the clinkers from the fires of cell processes or the ultimate effect of virus infections contracted in younger years. They may also be the result of destructive chemicals manufactured in the body.

There are lesions called "neurofibrillary tangles," twisted and pigmented nerve fibers in the brain. These tangles are more common in the elderly than in the young. They have been correlated with a decline in mental ability. Conversely, elderly people who have been outstanding intellectually, at autopsy show an absence of these tangles.

These observations are yet to be fully assessed. Even if such nerve pigments are damaging to the intellect, we only use half our brains anyway. When a stroke damages one side of the brain or half the brain is removed surgically or damaged by accident, we can learn to use the other half. We can remember things that happened in the past and we still remember how to do the things we have learned.

This has led, in part, to the belief that problems in learning in old age are more emotional than physical.

Everyone can remember how he learned something thoroughly for school and then when the teacher asked him to recite it, he was too nervous to remember. It's the same sort of thing that may happen to older people.

In Western society, we do not value the wisdom of the aged. In fact, we expect the elderly to fail in tests of intellect. When they are competing with younger people in tests, this creates anxiety in the aged and they do not perform as well as they are capable of doing with less stress. Memory, of course, is involved in learning.

When Canadian pioneer neurosurgeon Wilder Penfield stimulated a point in a patient's brain electrically, the patient recalled a whole flood of memories. Why? How are memories laid down? Why can't we recall certain things when we want to? Is anything truly forgotten?

Dr. Penfield believes in a sort of tape recorder located in some region of the brain, possibly the hippocampus, a sea-horsed-shaped section on the inner side of our brain. A special recording mechanism may enable an early thought sequence, which we know as recall, to pass again through our consciousness. Only those phenomena to which we have paid attention are preserved on the recorder. Sights, sounds, and observations that have not made an impression on our minds are not recorded.

But how are those impressions made? To find out how long it takes for a memory to become permanent, animals have been trained and then quickly anesthetized, shocked, or cooled, with the time between learning and interruption successively lengthened. If cooled too soon, trained hamsters could no longer find their way through a maze they had been taught to travel. Anesthetized mice no longer remembered how to avoid a shock. Obviously, these experiments demonstrate that memory takes time to form—but how much time? Is it stored on both sides of the brain? Can it be transferred from one side to the other? No one yet knows.

The discovery that memories are made by ribonucleic acid (RNA), the substance that does the legwork for the cell's mastermind, DNA, threw out the earlier theory that memories were electrically made (because the brain both transmits and receives electrical stimuli).

Why? When electrical impulses in the brain are interrupted, memory is not affected. But when an RNA inhibitor, such as the antibiotic puromycin, is injected, remembering becomes impossible. Furthermore, changes have been found in the amount and composition of the RNA in nerve cells during learning.

What does this mean to the young and old with poor memories? Untrained rats, when injected with an RNA-rich extract from the brains of well-trained donor rats, performed amazing tricks they had never been trained to do. And a Texas researcher believes in a "memory molecule." Georges Ungar, exploiting the fact that rats naturally like the dark, shocked them every time they went into the dark, until they became fearful of it. Then he extracted molecules from the brains of the rats frightened of the dark and injected them into the brains of unshocked rats. These native rats then showed the same distinct, unnatural fear of the dark. The doctor calls his memory molecule Scotophobin, from scotophobia, meaning "fear of the dark." Synthetic rat scotophobin injected into goldfish obtained similar results.

Human experiments with memory molecules are still some years away. Intravenous injections of RNA into patients with memory loss associated with hardening of the arteries or senility proved inconclusive. Whatever beneficial effects could be noticed lasted only as long as the period of administration of the RNA, which demonstrates that RNA may be no more than a nonspecific, or general, stimulant. However, interference with a natural stimulant, norepinephrine, which is manufactured by the adrenal glands, blocks memory in mice. Severe restrictions of amino acids essential for the manufacture of norepinephrine in man is already associated with memory defects.

Can anything be done now to improve failing memory?

Oxygen alone and oxygen under pressure has been tried in patients. Before and after receiving oxygen treatment, all the patients underwent psychological tests. Those who had breathed pure oxygen under pressure improved from 35 to 300 percent compared with controls who received no oxygen. The patients' behavior also improved. All those treated became more active, slept better, and asked for newspapers and magazines to read. And most important, they resumed old habits of caring for themselves. Several were able to go home on visits and four were able to remain at home. Such experiments with hyperbaric oxygen and brain function are continuing.

Memory medications also hold some promise. Magnesium pemoline administered to twenty-four senile and presenile patients resulted in "slight" to "considerable" memory improvement for those whose memories had not deteriorated too much.

Unfortunately sugar pills, thereafter, packed as much learning power as magnesium pemoline and hope quickly faded for a memory pill. But now there is renewed interest in the drug. A more refined form of the compound seems more powerful. In laboratory experiments it significantly enhances the learning ability in animals.

Another pill, one with a very different action, propanolol, is used in the treatment of irregular heart rhythms, and also blocks the effect of anxiety ("arousal"). During test-taking, the elderly release an enzyme that causes increased blood fats. Their blood fats during arousal were higher than that of young people under similar circumstances, and took longer to return to normal. When given propanolol, the release of blood fat was blocked in the elderly, and they did much better on mental tests. Why, exactly, no one knows.

The drug L-dopa, which has successfully freed many Parkinson's disease patients from the prisons of their own bodies and restored them to controlled movements, has been found to sharpen memory and heighten the intelligence of patients to whom it is administered.

A year's follow-up of eighteen patients with a median age of sixty-five years at Northwestern University Medical School showed that cognitive, conative, memory, and perceptual motor functioning improved for most patients. Verbal ability, information, and comprehension improved dramatically between the first test before they took L-dopa and the second test when they were judged to have achieved maximum benefit for their symptoms of parkinsonism.

Two other drugs are under testing. One is procaine, made famous by the Romanian gerontologist Ana Aslan as a youth drug. But American researchers know it as a monoamine oxidase inhibitor, which is a brain chemical associated with depression. Generally, when a person is depressed, he may have a poor memory and other manifestations of deteriorating mental functioning.

The other drug being tested is NPT-10381. It is derived from inosines, which are the breakdown products of the purine that forms in working muscles. Generally, inosines are used as flavor enhancers in food. They enhance protein and RNA synthesis in normal cells, which is food for memory, and interfere with protein synthesis and RNA production of viruses.

When given to old rats, their memory improved and they showed a greater aptitude for learning new things. Testing in humans is under way.

In still another chemical approach, senile patients benefited from anticoagulant drugs, drugs that thin the blood. By thinning the blood, the blood flow to the brain may be increased. Control patients in an old-age home continued to deteriorate rapidly mentally, whereas other patients in the home given anticoagulants showed only a slight decline.

However, mental decline in the aged may be due, in large part, from the deficiencies of vitamins B and C. The elderly, especially those who live alone, have very poor diets. When a group of senile patients suspected of vitamin deficiency were given massive doses of vitamins B and C, their abnormal mental condition rapidly improved, or their abnormality disappeared altogether.

No medication or oxygen treatment is going to affect mental functioning once the brain cells are gone. However, there are times when the brain cells are injured, or impaired, such as in a concussion or from high blood pressure. It is with temporarily injured or ill brain cells that medications and treatments can work to bring them back. But telling the difference between hopelessly dead cells and retrievable cells remains a problem for physicians.

Until there is a potent memory medication available, what can we do? Quite a lot. Just consider that stroke patients who lose the ability to talk, read, or understand speech can be taught to receive, interpret, and react to speech again.

The belief that firstborn and only children achieve more in life is attributed to their having been the center of attention when young; that they received more stimulation from adults than did younger siblings. Like using a muscle, their brains had more of a workout. It may have increased their very size and composition. Charles Darwin observed that domestic rabbits had smaller brains than wild rabbits. He reasoned that domestic rabbits had been fed and housed all their lives so, therefore, they did not need to develop their brains to survive in the wild.

Studies show in both humans and animals that intellectual stimulation can actually increase brain cells; that learning alters chemical activity and causes multiplication of cells in the cerebral cortex—the so-called thinking brain.

Therefore "teaching an old dog new tricks" may actually preserve and improve mental functioning and prolong life. A study of subjects over a twelve-year period did correlate maintenance of intellectual vigor with capacity to survive. Furthermore, aging business executives whose work required sharp intellect have little or no weakening of their nervous systems compared with aging production workers.

A system devised in 477 B.C. to improve memory function in stroke is still in use. Anyone can do it.

The system is based on the fact that memory is founded on associating what we want to remember with what we already know. The more vivid we can make visual associations, the better we can remember. The more concrete the item to be recalled, the more unusual or ridiculous the image created to associate it with, the easier it will be to remember.

Suppose you want to remember a shopping list of bread, eggs, flour, and orange juice. The first thing to do is picture a loaf of bread breaking open and an egg falling out. Then picture a pitcher of orange juice being poured into a hole in the flour bag. Each item is linked to the subsequent one via the ridiculous image. Stroke patients who used this method and who could not previously remember days and months were soon able to master the list of United States presidents.

Loss of intellectual abilities is not usually based on just one thing. It involves physical and psychological factors. Retirement, for instance, can be devastating to mental functioning.

But if we keep ourselves in as good working order as we keep our cars, that means eyeglasses and hearing aids if needed and medical control of blood pressure, heart disease, and other physical ills, if necessary, and enough rest and exercise and mental stimulation, then we will prevent or retard the brain's aging.

NIH's Dr. Nathan Shock summed it up when he said: "Oftentimes, what passes as aging is nothing more than atrophy, or disuse. This is especially true within the sphere of mental activities. A good dictum would be to learn something new every day even if it comes under the heading of useless information. We might well adapt the Boy Scout dictum of a 'good deed every day' to a 'new deed every day' for the maintenance of health and vigor in later years."

The multitalented Leonardo da Vinci said the same thing a long time ago: "Iron rusts from disuse, stagnant water loses its purity and in cold weather becomes frozen; even so does inaction sap the vigors of the mind."

Chapter 6

Aging Is Not Skin Deep

THE APPEARANCE OF THE first facial wrinkle can be traumatic, a sign for all the world to see that one is losing youth. And a wrinkle is just a single example of the changes that occur in skin as the years go by, changes that profoundly affect our entire being.

But, fortunately, there is much that can be done to prevent, correct, and cover up the skin's aging.

The skin performs many vital functions, including protecting our bodies against invasion by bacteria, against injury to the more sensitive tissues within, against the rays of the sun, and against the loss of moisture. It also serves as an extremely sensitive organ of perception because it contains thousands of pain, pressure, heat, and cold receptors.

Skin is generally soft and elastic in youth, varying in thickness from about one-fiftieth of an inch on the eyelids to as much as one-third of an inch on the palms and soles. But the thickness of the skin declines by about 50 percent between the ages of twenty and eighty due to changes in collagen—one of two major proteins that form structural, or "connective," tissues in the body. The other protein is elastin, and, as its name suggests, it is "stretchable."

Collagen represents 75 percent of the weight of the skin. It makes skin stronger than the other soft tissues, such as those of the intestines and liver. It is extremely tough, hard to bend, and, in fact, takes ten thousand times its own weight to stretch collagen. Elastin, on the other hand, which is just a small part of structural tissue, stretches easily. The outside ear is largely elastin, whereas collagen is a major component of ligaments, muscles, tendons, cartilage, the cornea of the eye, heart valves, and blood vessels.

The skin begins noticeably to lose some of its elasticity and flexibility during the late thirties, at the same time becoming thinner. This is because, it is believed, the collagen becomes more rigid, stiffening as its molecules form unbreakable bonds with each other, a process known as cross-linking. In virtually all animals tested, collagen becomes stiffer and stronger with age, and harder to dissolve. Experiments with collagen in rat tails and frog fingers indicate that the older the collagen, the harder it is to bend.

What causes the collagen to stiffen and form unbreakable bonds is still being debated. It may be a hormonal deficiency or some adverse chemical process at work.

Collagen is especially at work in a woman's skin, which, although romantically touted to be softer than a man's, is actually less stretchable and resilient, and it is thinner. This sex difference is attributed to an inborn tendency of a woman's skin collagen to form those cross-linked unbreakable bonds earlier than in a man's skin. Thus, the observation that a woman's skin ages more rapidly than a man's.

However, another theory is that the man's skin doesn't age as quickly as a woman's because a man shaves every day, constantly removing the dead cells of the outer layers and keeping new cells forming rapidly.

The skin is actually made up of three layers. The first, the deepest, the subcutaneous, contains fat, blood vessels, and nerves. It acts as a link between the tissues covering underlying muscle and bone and the next layer of skin, the dermis. It also serves as a mattress for the dermis and the epidermis, the two outer skins.

Although you'd never know it from reading some cosmetic ads, the submerged cutaneous skin is a large factor in wrinkling. As we age, its fat lobules diminish—perhaps from a hormonal deficiency—and consequently the mattress doesn't fully support the other skin covers. Furthermore, the loss of underlying fat means a loss of the insulation that helps keep the body temperature constant. Subcutaneous fat also serves as a cushion against injury. Therefore, its loss contributes to the difficulty older people have in maintaining body temperature, and explains why older people are prone to skin sores at points of pressure.

The middle layer of skin, the dermis, sometimes called the true skin, varies in thickness in different parts of the body. It contains blood vessels, nerves, nerve receptors, hair follicles, sweat glands, and oil glands.

A sweat gland begin as a coil located in the dermis and winds its way upward to the skin's surface, where a pore is formed. It releases a watery liquid that contains small amounts of salts and other materials.

The oil glands, also in the dermis, are found in every area of the skin, except the palms, soles, fingernails, and toenails. They are usually most numerous around the nose, cheeks, mouth, and chin.

Both sweat and sebum, the product of the oil glands, are delivered to the skin surface by thousands of glands. On the surface they mix together, and the oil of the sebum combines with the water of the sweat to form an emulsion. The result of this most natural "cosmetic" is a soft, pliable skin surface.

As we age, the sweat and oil glands atrophy—dramatically in women after the menopause and generally much sooner in women than in men. This creates a dry, uncomfortable, itching skin. And if no moisture or oil is added, we can expect fissures, or cracks, which are painful, and fine wrinkles.

The loss of sweat glands affects our ability to adjust to temperature change just as much as does the loss of subcutaneous fat, though differently. The water that sweat glands release cools the body by evaporation, an action controlled by a heat regulator in the brain. As the brain ages and the sweat glands diminish, it becomes harder for the body to adjust to heat.

Oil gland loss, too, is critical to the health of the skin because it is a natural protector against skin problems, including skin tumors and calluses.

With aging, it is the increased fragility of the blood vessels in the dermal and subcutaneous layers that causes our skin to turn black and blue. Changes in the blood vessels in the skin may also cause bulges or so-called varicose veins. Such broken blood vessels, particularly in the legs, may occur as early as thirty years in areas of greatest strain—the outer surface of the mid-thighs, just below the knees, and around the ankles. Their only significance usually is cosmetic; the color often imitates bruises. Some researchers believe the breaks may result from the blockage of circulation by garters or tight girdles, or by keeping the legs crossed too long, or standing for an extended time.

A physician should be consulted if there is any physical discomfort associated with the blemish or if such broken vessels occur on the trunk or on the face. These may be caused by serious disorders and not aging skin.

The top layer of skin, the epidermis, is sometimes called the "horny layer" because it is made up of scales that are actually dead skin cells. These are the cells that fall off as we move about or soak off when we bathe. However, the horny layer is constantly being replaced by cells pushed to the surface as new cells are formed in the deeper skin layers, a process that takes from two weeks to about a month. Since the epidermis is constantly being renewed, some people claim that it is forever young.

In the deeper layers of the skin where new cells are constantly being formed, there is also a coloring—melanin—which is designed to prevent the more dangerous rays of the sun from damaging tissue. Melanin also influences skin color. The more of it you have, the darker your skin. Blacks have the most. As we age, it builds up in our skin, generally, but more particularly in spots.

Those pigment freckles known as "age," or "liver," spots consist of melanin. They become more prevalent as we pass from the fourth to the fifth and sixth decades of life. As the accumulation of melanin spots increases, so do wartlike growths known as seborrheic keratoses, which have been linked to malfunctioning of the sweat glands, causing seborrhea, Seborrhea is a condition characterized by excessive secretion of sebum or an alteration in its quality, resulting in an oily coating, crusts, or scales on the skin.

Independent of melanin, the horny layer of the skin gets thicker, while the underlying layers of the skin get thinner. This results in a reduction of the working layers of the skin to a fraction of their former thickness, while the outer layer becomes both thicker and harder, accentuating lines and wrinkles. Added to the melanin buildup over the years, we get a leathery wrinkled, darkened skin.

As we grow old, not only does the appearance of our skin change, its ability to heal itself does also. The time necessary for the self-repair of a skin wound almost doubles between the ages of twenty and forty years.

How can we limit the changes that take place in the three layers of the skin? And can anything be done to prevent such changes?

The first thing that can be done is simply to stay out of the sun as much as possible. Sun-damaged skin becomes dry, coarse, leathery, loose, and wrinkled. Even infrequent sunning adds up because all radiation, even from long-past exposure, is cumulative in this effect.

Sun-induced aging begins early in life. Microscopic changes were detected in 20 percent of a group of children under ten years of age. And studies have shown that four out of five teen-agers have sun-damaged skin and that the amount of damage increases steadily with age and exposure, even without actual sunburn.

If you are light-complexioned, a freckled redhead, a blue-eyed blond, you are more susceptible to the rays of the sun than dark-haired people. Blacks are least affected, but they are not totally exempt from sun damage.

When a normal person has been mildly overexposed to the sun, the skin may turn red six to twelve hours after exposure, reaching its peak in about twenty-four hours. Whereas, a mild sunburn generally results in tanned skin, a severe sunburn results in blistering, pain, sickness, and sometimes death. Even the small doses of sunlight that strike the skin daily cause the skin to age. Deliberate sunbathing just speeds up the process; it irreversibly damages the skin.

The teen-aged girl who bakes in the sun each year to attain a glorious tan may find that when she is forty years old, her skin will appear fifty-five to sixty years old. The facial skin of many older persons has marked degenerative changes, whereas the parts of their skin not exposed to sunlight have healthy tissue and the elastic fibers of young skin.

Look at your buttocks, if you are not a bikini wearer. The skin will be much younger in appearance than the skin on your face. As Benjamin Franklin once observed, perhaps not quite accurately, put a barrel over the head and shoulders of a woman and you cannot tell her age.

Because the sun is so obviously bad for skin, some dermatologists have tried to change the scientific name for aging skin—from "Senile Elastosis" to "Solar Elastosis," meaning loss of elasticity due to sunlight.

Why sunlight damages skin is not quite clear, but it may be due to the sun's ability to mutate or foul up the DNA, the genetic code of skin cells. If sun-damaged skin cannot be rejuvenated, then something basic has been affected, a University of Pennsylvania dermatologist reasons.

Dr. Albert Kligman took a piece of skin from the sun-exposed area of the forearm of eighteen persons in an old-age home and transplanted it to their abdomens. Skin from their abdomens was then transplanted to their forearms.

Of course, the darker forearm skin grafts were strikingly contrasted against the surrounding lighter abdominal skin, and remained tan for four years, despite the absence of sun exposure. Conversely, the white abdominal skin transplanted to the forearm remained as pale squares thriving in the midst of the darker sun-damaged skin.

This was proof for Dr. Kligman that sun-damaged skin cells undergo permanent fundamental alterations in their genetic material.

So, if you wish to retard the aging of your skin, stay out of the sun as much as possible, particularly between noon and three o'clock when the sun's rays are strongest. If you must go in the sun, wear a sun-screen lotion that will protect your skin.

What else can you do? If you smoke, give it up. If you don't smoke, don't start. In a study by a California internist, an examination of some 1,100 subjects showed a strong association between prolonged smoking and "crow's feet," wrinkles around the eyes. Longtime smokers at the age of fifty had the crow's feet of seventy-year-olds. Those who had smoked heavily during youth—before wrinkling occurs—and had given it up, still had deeper crow's feet at fifty years than those who never smoked.

You can keep your skin from drying out too much by limiting your exposure to air conditioning and nonhumidified household heating systems. Both remove moisture from the air and consequently from your skin.

Detergents, household cleansers, and soap can also dry the skin, and older people should use them sparingly. In fact, many dermatologists suggest that anyone past forty-five years cut down on bathing to preserve the natural body oils, and that cleansing cream be substituted for soaps or detergents to cleanse the skin.

Long before Cleopatra met Antony, women have been creaming their skins in an effort to keep them soft and supple. Lubricating the skin, most dermatologists agree, is worthwhile. As we age and the glands of the skin begin to decrease their activity and there is insufficient sebum to keep the skin as soft as in the teen years, external emollients provide part of the oil the skin needs. The only qualification is that whether you use cooking oil or expensive commercial creams, the results are the same.

Aging skin has been compared to an old girdle that has lost its elasticity. No amount of massage or chemicals will restore an old girdle. But you can take care of that girdle so that it doesn't wear out too fast. You can do the same thing for your skin. An oily substance will protect your skin from the elements and retard evaporation of its own moisture. Therefore, it will retard drying and wrinkling of the skin, but the addition of exotic ingredients such as placenta extract or turtle oil do nothing more than raise the cost of the product. And when it comes to wrinkles, there are no smooth turtles. External oils cannot put moisture in despite such claims by advertisers.

As for the addition of estrogen hormone to facial cream, here it does no more than raise the cost of the product. In experiments with two identical creams, except that one contained estrogen, results were the same; there was no appreciable difference in the effects of the creams on the skin. However, the ordinary oil contained in both creams did have a beneficial effect on the skin.

This is not to say that hormones cannot be used to retard aging of the skin. As the chapter on hormones described, supplementary estrogen after menopause does help to keep the skin supple and healthy. And hormone creams are used topically in the vaginal area to combat dry, thin skin there. But, of course, the use of hormones should be controlled by a physician.

What can be done about the freckles known as "age spots"?

Vitamin E, which is an antioxidant and a suspected hormone activator, may be useful in preventing such spots, although its use in this respect is still controversial. If you look at rancid fat, you see brown spots. This is what is believed to happen in the body, and those brown spots in the skin are the result of "rancid" body fat. Vitamin E prevents such rancidity in fat and is used as an antioxidant in certain food products containing fats and oils. The National Academy of Sciences' Food and Nutrition Board set minimum daily requirements for vitamin E at thirty international units for adults. However, no one has proved or disproved vitamin E's part in preventing age freckles.

Avoiding the use of perfume when you go out in the sun may prevent certain types of brown spots known as berloque dermatitis. These spots are caused by the oil of bergamot contained in many perfumes. It reacts on the skin of susceptible people during exposure to sunlight, causing permanent discoloration.

Once brown spots occur, other than bleaching creams on

the market to lighten them and makeup, of course, to hide them, doctors have had some success in reducing age pigments with chemical surgery called face peeling, which you will read about later in this chapter.

Another skin coloring problem concerns small blood vessels that begin to show on the nose and spread over the face. Called telangiectasia (*telos* meaning "end," *angeion* meaning "vessel," and ectasis referring to "stretching out"), they appear as red, weblike blemishes. There are many causes of such telangiectasia including heredity, excessive exposure to sunlight, liver damage, and a skin disease called rosacea. Only a physician can make the diagnosis. Telangiectasia can be prevented, in some instances, depending upon the cause of the condition, by avoiding exposure to cold, wind, sun, and heat, or any dramatic change in temperature. Also, elimination of very hot or highly spiced foods and beverages from the diet helps prevent the red, weblike blemishes.

Whereas cosmetic defect caused by telangiectasia can be minimized by makeup if permanent removal is desirable, a physician uses an electric needle or dry ice to destroy the lesions.

Other cosmetic imperfections that occur frequently in aging skin include senile keratose, (precancerous lesions), common warts, and calluses. They can easily be removed by electrosurgery (burning with current), freezing, chemical surgery, or by conventional scalpel surgery.

For the more ambitious, there is plastic surgery. At one time surgery to ease the outer signs of aging was reserved for well-to-do people and those in the public eye. But it was done surreptitiously, in the manner of an illegal abortion.

Today both men and women in increasing numbers are undergoing cosmetic surgery. The average female patient is between forty and sixty and most frequently is a housewife. The average male tends to be a salesman, business executive, or professional who deals constantly with people in close contact.

The most common skin problems that drive aging men to the plastic surgeon are sagging eyelids, the frown between the eyebrows, and the "turkey gobbler" neck. Laugh lines, under-the-eye pouches, and wrinkled skin under the chin are the most frequent symptoms that send older women to the plastic surgeon.

There is also so-called sagging face, caused by a "relaxation" of the skin. It is called "cutis laxa," or dermatolysis, often the unexpected, dramatic result of a successful reducing diet. Doctors warn that if you want to take off a lot of weight, do so while your skin is still young and elastic enough to snap into place after underlying fat has been removed through weight loss.

The folds of skin drooping about the cheeks and neck can be removed today only by surgery called "facial dermatoplasty," or face-lifting. It is a major operation, requiring at least two days in the hospital and three or four weeks of recovery.

Before performing any plastic surgery for "age signs," the plastic surgeon will evaluate or have a psychiatrist evaluate why the person wants a face-lift. If the reasons are sound and a face-lift would be genuinely beneficial, the surgeon will carefully chart the location of the incisions in advance. He will make sure they are hidden in the natural folds above and around the ears or in the hair behind the ears.

The basic face-lift involves lifting the skin, the sagging muscles, and the connective tissue. Local anesthesia is usually used because it is safer and causes less bleeding. The skin and muscle are pulled above the cheekbones and fastened near the hairline or ears. Excess skin—as much as two inches all around —is then snipped off.

A pressure dressing is applied.

The face-lift takes about two hours on the operating table and costs from $1,500 to $2,000, a sum not covered by most health insurance policies.

The so-called "mini" face-lift is done in a physician's office. Under local anesthesia, a triangle of skin is cut out above the temple hairline on both sides of the head. Then the edges of the skin are sewn together, "lifting" the upper part of the face. The results may be more gratifying psychologically than physically since the skin can only be slightly tightened in the middle and upper third of the face.

Wrinkling of the skin, which is different from "cutis laxa," is called "rhytidosis." Though the former may produce the later, the treatment of each is different.

For removal of wrinkles, a physician—and it should be only a physician although there are other operators in the field—uses either a "chemical face peel" or "dermabrasion."

Face peeling is a procedure that destroys living tissue by the action of caustic chemicals such as phenol or trichloroacetic acid. It was originally designed to remove small, benign lesions. However, it was found to erase wrinkles.

During a face peel a liquid chemical is applied and the entire face is covered with a waterproof adhesive tape, leaving only the eyes and mouth and nose exposed. After forty-eight hours, the tape is peeled off under anesthetic, and the burned skin comes with it. The patient returns home in five to seven days, and in about twenty-eight days new skin is regenerated. The elasticity of the skin may be improved with a decrease in freckles and fine to moderate wrinkles. In the early weeks after treatment, improvement is dramatic because of the residual swelling of the skin. However, after three or four months, improvement is less marked, although still apparent. The average fee is $750. The best candidates are light-skinned people because those with darker skin tend to show the lines of chemical bleach demarcation. There are also potential side effects such as scarring and dark spots.

In dermabrasion the skin is frozen and a rapidly rotating brush is stroked across the face to remove the upper layers of skin down to the level of the wrinkles. The procedure can also be done by hand, using sandpaper. Swelling and extensive crusting develop in the first twenty-four to forty-eight hours; then the crusts are shed in about two weeks, leaving the skin underneath a little more pink than before. The skin returns to a normal color within a few weeks.

Dermabrasion can be done in several sessions in a physician's office. The cost depends upon several factors, including the size of the area to be treated. Generally, the price ranges between $200 and $750.

A combination or each alone of chemical peel and dermabrasion may be used with a face-lift.

Another surgical technique that may be necessary even in young people is blepharoplasty, the removal of skin from the eyelids and from below the eye. Bags under the eyes, or drooping lids, result from heredity as well as age. There are three basic conditions: The first is the rumpled skin that is usually the result of frequent bouts of swelling from allergy or kidney problems or some other cause; the second is extra, stretched skin of the upper eyelid, which may cause the lid to droop; the third and most common is due to fat deposits, which cause baggy eyelids and pouches under the eyes.

For a blepharoplasty, the skin around the eye is marked before surgery so that the surgeon knows exactly how much skin to remove. Performed at the hospital under local anesthesia, an incision is made through the muscles around the eyes, and underlying excess fat is removed. An S-shaped section of skin is removed and the remaining skin is pulled tight. The eye lift takes about an hour. Dressings are applied and four days after surgery, they are removed, the stitches taken out, and the patient sent home. The cost is about $500 to $1,200. Plastic surgeons warn about using false eyelashes too soon after the operation because they can stretch the scars.

Still another technique for removing wrinkles on both the face and hands involves the injection of a plastic substance—silicone—under the skin to fill out the wrinkles. Small amounts of the plastic are injected by a thin needle deep under the wrinkles. There have been some poor results, including plastic floating throughout the body. The procedures are now being done experimentally only by a few doctors with the permission of the United States Food and Drug Administration.

Sagging breasts and small breasts may also be shaped up with silicone implants. These are soft, fluid-filled bags that are on the market and freely accessible to plastic surgeons and approved as safe by the FDA. In augmenting the breast, the patient is placed in a sitting position. At the crease between the breasts, an incision is made. While the patient is in a prone position, the implant is inserted through the incision. Strenuous exercise is not permitted for six weeks until the implant is firmly in place.

When breasts are too large or sagging, the nipple is removed, the breast is partially amputated and contoured, and a new site for the nipple is made. The grafted nipple regains sensitivity and has a normal appearance, but the possibility of breast feeding a child is, of course, eliminated.

Surgery can also correct other signs of age. There are abdominal lifts, arm, hips, and thigh lifts. Relaxed, flabby abdomens and flabby arms and thighs may evolve with age or loss of weight, or because of heredity. Such flab, however, is most often seen in persons who lose weight in middle age when the skin can no longer shrink and contract to take up the slack. The overabundance of relaxed skin and fat is removed with shallow incisions to avoid touching the muscle or major blood vessels. For example, when the fat roll of the lower abdomen is removed, the horizontal incision is so slight that the scar is easily hidden by underwear or a bathing suit. The muscles of the abdomen may also be tightened during the procedure and if a hernia is present, that too will be repaired. The belly button, if removed during surgery, will be sewn back in its proper place.

A young woman with multiple pregnancies also may benefit from such an abdominal operation because her muscles may have been stretched beyond the point of no return.

For the arm lift, the incision is made along the inside and back of the upper arm, from just above the elbow to the armpit.

For the thighs, the incision is usually made from the side of the hips, crossing the buttocks, removing the fat and hoisting up the thighs and buttocks.

All plastic surgery to remove signs of age should not be taken lightly. It is expensive, usually uncompensated by health insurance, and should be performed only when absolutely necessary.

What is the ideal age for surgical removal of the signs of

aging of the skin? Most doctors believe it is between forty-five and fifty-five years, but some will do persons thirty-five years or younger, if necessary. There is no age limit set at the other end, as long as the person's health permits. Such techniques can remove ten to twenty years from a person's face and body. How long will the results last? Five to ten years, provided the recipient stays away from too much sun and sufficiently lubricates the skin and does not overeat.

A much easier sign of aging to correct, though artificially, is the graying of hair. However, research into its causes continues. There are several types of hair and all of them are part of the skin. Hairs range in texture from the soft, almost imperceptible hair of the forehead to the long hairs of the scalp and the short, stiff hairs on the eyelids. Hair appears on all parts of the skin except the palms and soles.

Products to cover gray have always been the biggest money-makers in the hair cosmetic business. And the revenue is increasing all the time as more men join women in hiding this sign of aging.

Obvious gray hair is present at about thirty-five years in the average person, but can appear as early as twenty years and as late as fifty. In the middle thirties the amount of gray hair is rarely so great that brunettes, blonds, and redheads lose their identity. But, by the middle or late forties gray often predominates to a point where one is identified as "gray-haired."

The process of hair graying is usually slow but unrelenting. It begins at the temples and extends over the entire head. Occasionally, the process slows down after the temple hairs turn gray. Some people have a white forelock, but it is not the result of aging but of an inherited dominant trait usually present at birth.

Hair turning white overnight is often described as the result of a severe emotional shock. Among the most famous alleged cases are those of Marie Antoinette and Sir Thomas More. Their hair supposedly turned white the night before their executions. However, there has never been a scientifically proved case of hair turning white overnight. The physical properties of hair make this unlikely. Hair is literally dead from scalp to tip.

Below the skin surface, hair is constantly being renewed. Each hair remains on the head for two to six years, and then falls out—at the rate of about sixty a day. Though such hairs are replaced by new hair sprouts from the same bulb, hair grows slowly, one-half inch a month. Healthy hair depends on a delicate balance of proteins within the hair shaft and oils on the outside of it.

A number of conditions may bring on early appearing or rapidly graying hair. Gray hair has been observed in infants with dietary deficiencies, over or under activity of the thyroid gland, and other disturbances of hormone function. Scalp troubles bring on early gray hair, and injury or disease of the nervous system sometimes causes graying patterns. Paralysis on one side of the body may cause loss of hair color on the affected side. Premature graying can follow a severe illness such as typhus, malaria, or influenza. No one knows why.

As hair grays it also changes texture. It becomes thicker and coarser. In men this occurs particularly in the nose and ears. Women may develop coarse hair on the lips and cheeks.

Can gray hair be returned to its original color? No, when graying is part of normal aging. Perhaps, when it results from disease.

There is little doubt in the minds of scientists, however, that when they fully understand the hormonal or other chemical changes that cause hair to lose its color, they will be able to prevent it or reverse it.

As we age, the hair grows more slowly, and the hair bulbs begin to shrivel. A burgeoning bald spot may appear on the top of the head, another of the outward signs of aging in a large percentage of men and a smaller percentage of women.

For some unexplained reason, men apparently are losing their hair at an earlier age than in previous generations. Dermatologists report that twenty years ago if a man began losing his hair before the age of twenty-six years, it was premature. Now they see many boys of eighteen and nineteen years who are going bald.

Some specialists believe that earlier balding is part of evolution and that someday all men will be bald. But endocrinologists maintain baldness is due to an increase in the male hormone, testosterone. The more a man has, the balder he gets. Yet, there has been limited success in regrowing hair by treating the scalp with testosterone. A fuzz has appeared but physicians question the possibility of adverse systemic effects from testosterone.

Whereas many men may resent their loss of hair, when a woman begins to bald, the results can be tragic, and their numbers are increasing. It may be because women are becoming more masculine. When given male hormones, women show a hair-growth increase on their bodies and a decrease on their heads. The pressures on women today could be stimulating the adrenal cortex, the outer layer of the adrenal gland, which is the body's major stress organ to produce more male hormone, with the resultant masculinizing effects.

Heredity factors also account for hair loss. A woman, for example, with sparse, thinning hair would have had a mother or grandmother with the same condition. Many factors may cause a woman's hair to thin out before she reaches the age of forty or even thirty, but this early type of hair loss is usually temporary, and should not be cause for alarm. Among the causes of this type of hair fallout are pregnancy, certain medicines, illnesses accompanied by high fever, and molting periods, which set no patterns. Other factors that have been implicated, but which are not proved causes of diffuse hair loss, include tight rollers, cheap hair dyes, ponytail hair styles, emotional upsets, and air pollution.

For those who prefer a more natural approach than a wig or toupee, there has been limited success with hair transplants. Tiny plugs of hair are taken from the back and side of the head and implanted on the top of the head. The procedure is based on the fact that the hair-bearing scalp, when transplanted from one area to another, retains its characteristics for hair growth.

Usually performed in a physician's office, the patient is placed face down. A local anesthetic is injected and a small instrument, about ⅛ inch in diameter connected to a motor-driven drill, punches out a small section of skin bearing hair. About forty to fifty grafts are taken in an hour and the donor wounds are closed, if necessary. Then holes are punched in the bald area and the grafts are implanted in the spaces, which are about four to five millimeters apart. An interesting aspect of hair grafts is that transplanted hair to the front would go gray at the same time it would have if left on the back.

With a successful transplant procedure, a person looks as if he has just begun to go bald. But the process is long and expensive, varying in cost from about $5 a plug to $25. Six or seven treatments of forty to sixty grafts each may be required.

A technique of weaving additional hair with sparse hair is also performed. It is done by laymen and is less expensive, but also less permanent. The person with woven hair can swim and do almost anything that is done with natural hair, since no glue is involved and the false hair is firmly anchored.

In addition to the epidermis and the hair, there is still another kind of skin—fingernails and toenails. Though hair and nails don't resemble each other, both have many things in common. They have their beginnings deep inside the skin, both can be cut and trimmed without pain as long as the attachment to the skin is not disturbed, and both are dependent upon the body for nourishment and growth.

While hair grows in a single shaft, nails grow as a slightly curved surface. And nails don't carry any inherited difference in color and curl. Yet, both nails and hair are made of dead protein—keratin. However, hair is flexible and nails are firm.

Nails grow about one millimeter per week at age twenty and slow to 0.5 millimeter per week at age eighty. This is much slower at all times than hair but fast enough to replace worn-out nail tips. However, since we no longer use our nails as weapons, as our ancestors did, we have to trim them or we would be unable to use our fingers effectively.

The visible portion of the nail is called the nail plate. The structure of the nail plate itself, as well as its atttachment to the underlying tissue, determines the color of the nail. At the base of each nail, where it disappears under the cuticle, is a small arc of lighter color, where the nail is manufacturing nutrients into new nail cells. This area is called the lunula. Cells in the lunula continue to undergo keratinization, and as the nail grows out from the area, the cells become fully hardened. If a nail is torn off completely or dissolved in a powerful acid, this regeneration plant will, if not damaged beyond repair, completely build a new nail in three to four months.

Trauma directly to the nail bed may result in the formation of a temporary blood clot, followed by a ridge across the nail that will eventually grow out. However, ridging due to severe damage to the nail bed may not disappear but be constantly reproduced by the damaged mechanism. As we age, the nails become more ridged and thicker, probably because of previous damage sustained by the lunula.

Skin diseases at or near the nail bed are by far the most common cause of distorted nail growth. Any inflammation involving the area around the nail bed may cause distortion of the nail. The origin of the nail extends almost as far back under the skin as the last finger joint. Therefore, inflammation of the joint, such as caused by arthritis, can lead to fingernail deformities.

Psoriasis, ringworm, chemical or physical injury, or injury to the nerves supplying this area will cause variations in keratin production. Systemic diseases that interfere with the blood supply to the extremities, such as pneumonia, will also cause similar changes in nail growth.

Any changes and problems in the cells that form the nail may be reflected by changes in the nail's appearance. A previous injury, even a minor one, may lead to grooving and splitting.

The best preventative for splitting and peeling nails is to cut the nails short so that they do not catch against various objects. Some studies indicate improvement after daily doses of gelatin. Creams and oils for nails may counteract surface drying but will not cure brittle nails. To prevent brittle nails, wear rubber gloves with cotton linings whenever possible when doing wet household or work chores.

Thickening of the nails is seen almost always on the toes. The chief causes, aside from hereditary factors that promote overproduction of keratin, are failure to keep toenails trimmed and the wearing of tight shoes that do not allow nails to grow outward. This condition is more common in males than females, probably because women trim their toenails more often. In the rare cases where thickened fingernails occur, it is usually due to work that requires frequent picking up of small objects with the nails or repeated injury to the hands of the type suffered by carpenters and other workmen. In such cases the body protects itself by producing a thicker shield of keratin.

Discolored nails are fairly common and the staining may arise from the nicotine in tobacco, chemicals used at work, or certain drugs. Any form of stress, such as physical injury, may turn nails blue black or gray. Such stains may be prevented by protecting the hands from the offending chemicals.

In the matter of nails, as with hair and skin, continued research with hormones and their ultimate control will one day enable us to arrest and reverse the aging process.

Chapter 7

The Die in Diet

IF YOU CAN CONTROL your diet, you can significantly control your aging. You not only are what you eat—you age by what you eat.

Evidence points to overnutrition as the culprit that shortens man's life-span. For every pound of fat above normal, there must be an expanded system of blood vessels, which in turn requires one's heart to pump extra gallons of blood over longer distances. The extra fat puts an extra burden on the heart.

Not only the heart is affected. The old saying that the longer the belt line, the shorter the lifeline is borne out by many studies. A study of normal and overweight East Germans showed that the overweight developed age-associated degenerative diseases such as heart attacks, cancer, and high blood pressure ten years earlier than their slimmer counterparts. For Americans 30 percent over their normal weight, the death rate increases 40 percent.

The life-shortening effect of overweight was demonstrated in animals as far back as 1927 when Dr. Clive McCay of Cornell University produced his now classic experiments. He gave rats an adequate amount of vitamins, minerals, and protein in their food but greatly reduced the number of calories. He not only slowed down their rate of maturing but also extended their life-span. After a thousand days, the underfed rats still looked young whereas fellow rats on the normal, calorie-filled diet did not survive more than 965 days. Some of the "starved" rats survived 1,400 days.

Similar results were gained in more recent dietary experiments with rotifers, a tiny one thousand-cell aquatic animal that reproduces without help from the opposite sex; this assures the same genetic program in each generation of rotifer.

When the tiny animals were raised in an environment of thirty-five degrees Centigrade, they lived only eighteen days. When the environmental temperature was reducd to a low of twenty-five degrees, they survived thirty-four days. When their food intake was cut roughly in half, their life-span increased to fifty-five days.

There appeared to be two separate timetables for aging in the rotifer—one for early life and another for late life. Rotifers raised in a lower temperature gained a longer life-span after egg-laying ceased, while those whose diets were restricted gained the time during the fertile period. Regardless of the environmental conditions, all rotifers laid approximately forty eggs. However, those rotifers whose life-span was increased by dietary restriction took longer to lay the forty eggs.

The conclusion? That the activity of the enzymes—the workhorses of the cell that carry out the manufacturing processes—may be the "expression of program," the catalysts that cause events to happen. By manipulating the environment and the diet, one can affect the activity of the enzymes and thus ultimately the life-span of the body.

In the early life of the rotifer, the enzymes can be markedly influenced by diet but not apparently by temperature. In the second part of the program, the later part of life, the enzymes are apparently altered by temperature but not by nutrition.

How does this research apply to human beings?

Growing evidence suggests that we may be giving our children too much nutrition too soon. Obesity in many children and adults may have its origin in infancy. Infants tend to regulate their food intake by volume rather than by nutritional content. Therefore, they often consume inordinate quantities of formulas highly concentrated in calories and protein. This unconscious gluttony may stimulate into existence excessive numbers of fat storage cells and, thereby, trigger in many infants a genetic predisposition to overweight that can plague them throughout adulthood and shorten their lives.

We also are possibly speeding up the programming of children's enzymes and thus ultimately cutting short their potential life-span.

One effect of super-nutrition is quite clear to everyone. Children are getting bigger faster. The average height of a ten-year-old American boy has increased about half an inch per decade. Over the past ninety years, the rise in the average weight for boys six to eleven years has been 15 to 30 percent. Thus, a boy who was ten years old in 1875 might have been only 50 percent through his growth cycle, whereas a boy in the mid-1960s might have been 60 to 65 percent mature.

In 1877 a fourteen-year-old high-school boy averaged 4 feet 7½ inches in height and weighed eighty-seven pounds. Today's fourteen-year-old is six inches taller and thirty pounds heavier.

And we're growing them bigger all the time. When government researchers recently checked a group of eighteen- to seventy-nine-year-olds, they found the men averaged seven pounds heavier and the women eleven pounds heavier than a similar group studied only seven years ago.

In 1900 less than 4 percent of American women grew to 5 feet 7 inches. Today at least 18 percent of the women between ages twenty and twenty-nine are that tall—or taller. In the same period fewer than four out of one hundred men reached six feet. Now more than twenty-five out of one hundred are six feet or more.

Why are Americans reaching new heights?

Genetic mixing is one answer. The tall and the short are marrying and producing bigger children. Environment is a factor. This includes change of climate and perhaps longer periods of light thanks to artificial lighting; experiments with plants and animals show that light influences growth.

The greatest factor influencing growth, however, is apparently nutrition. We don't wait anymore for babies to get a single tooth. We feed them strained meat, sometimes within days of birth. Meat is high in proteins, large molecules in which various amino acids, the basic building blocks of life, are linked together in long, precise sequences.

The effects of super-nutrition are perhaps most dramatic in Japan. Japanese children born after World War II are consuming a diet richer in protein by 20 percent. When they reach school, these children can no longer fit into the school desks used by their parents.

Does this mean that longevity will be cut because American and Japanese children are literally being forced to "grow up too fast?"

Although dietary-restriction experiments have not really been done on man, there is every reason to believe that the rotifer phenomenon would work as well with humans. Under laboratory conditions, just this effect was shown in the daphnia, the fruit fly, the mouse, and the rat, as well as the rotifer. So why should man be different?

How would we go about restricting nutrition and extending life in humans?

One way, in animals, is to give just half of what the subject would like to eat and restricted to only 20 to 25 percent protein.

Another way is to give the animal as much as it wants to eat, but reduce the amount of protein to 4 to 8 percent.

With both diets, animals live longer.

What about people, especially those who are undernourished from the beginning because they can't afford a generous diet?

The most common nutritional deficiency in the world caused by a chronic lack of protein in the diet is kwashiorkor. Originally identified in Ghana in 1960, kwashiorkor is rampant in most developing nations. Children with this disease suffer severe growth retardation, vulnerability to illness, swelling of the abdomen with water, and marked apathy. Kwashiorkor patients are so apathetic that a treated youngster who smiles is considered on the road to recovery.

Whereas kwashiorkor is extreme protein deficiency, a little protein deficiency, according to our standards, may be beneficial. In Czechoslovakia the very old reported experiencing a very modest or insufficient diet during their childhood school days. A deficiency in animal protein or fat was typical and there was a lack of fancy foodstuffs with so-called empty calories.

However, with kwashiorkor, there are multiple deficiency problems, not just low protein. But there are difficulties in choosing a good diet for humans. Animals in a laboratory live in a stress-free environment—in a glass cage. They are not subject to the same stresses as man throughout his life-span.

But with dietary restriction, in reducing the amount of protein, we slow down protein synthesis. As a result, we may be minimizing the use of the genetic code and thereby limiting the readout of lethal genes or protecting the genes from damage.

There are known mass dietary experiments, though unintentional, on humans. These occurred in Israel. The influx of Oriental (Yemenite) Jews, who had a different diet from the European Jews, presented an excellent living laboratory for the study of nutrition and its effect on health.

These Yemenites who came to Israel more than thirty years ago had zero diabetes compared to a rate of 3.5 per 1,000 for their European brethren in Israel. The Yemenites also had less cancer of the lung, 5 per 100,000 compared to 16 per 100,000. And the Yemenites were heavy smokers.

Yet, today, Yemenite Israelis have the same heart attack and cancer rate as European Israelis.

Among reasons given for the changes are mental stress, work, and eating habits.

The Yemenite's customary source of carbohydrate from bread was replaced by sugar, the European source. They put on weight and as Israeli and other scientists have observed, thin people are less likely to get cancer.

In Ireland an examination of insurance records for men

between 1887 and 1921 also showed a positive correlation between the incidence of cancer of all types and increasing body weight. Doctors in Minnesota and in Australia have correlated the fact that the malnourished are less susceptible to cancer than the well fed. In human beings regression or marked slowing in the spread of local tumors and cancer cells has followed diets deficient in essential amino acids such as phenylalanine and tyrosine. Leukemia, Hodgkin's disease, and cancer of the uterus have also regressed in response to certain dietary restrictions.

How can diet affect cancer in this way? Scientists speculate that such restrictions limit the nutriments necessary for malignant cell proliferation, literally starving certain cancers. They also believe that undernutrition somehow stimulates the body's own immunologic system. Of course, too much starvation can make people more susceptible to infection.

There are many paradoxes and intriguing clues in the mystery of diet and aging. Much of the mystery is believed to concern free radicals. Free radicals are highly electrically charged pieces of molecules that are born during the course of chemical reactions. Free radical reactions are commonplace. They occur in the automobile engine when oxygen reacts with gasoline; in smog formation; and when fat such as butter or cholesterol combines with oxygen and becomes rancid. Free radicals are also believed to occur when we eat more than our bodies can use.

Free radicals, to put it more picturesquely, occur when two constables meet and shake hands and allow a maniac in their charge to escape. Some free radical maniacs are more dangerous than others. Once a free radical escapes, it's not recoverable. For instance, you can't take the carbon dioxide and water coming from an automobile exhaust and change it back into the original gasoline and oxygen.

Evidence seems to be mounting implicating free radical reactions in the pathogenesis of major age-associated diseases such as cancer, atherosclerosis, and high blood pressure. Free radicals caused by such things as X rays and nuclear radiation have been implicated in tumor development.

Free radicals are formed in the so-called low cholesterol diet, which is high in unsaturated fats (usually vegetable fats that are liquid at room temperature). Such a diet may contribute to the aging process because these fats combine more readily with oxygen than saturated, animal fats, which are hard at room temperature.

Ironically, the polyunsaturated diet recommended by the American Heart Association, therefore, may have just the opposite effect than intended. The AHA recommends saturated fats such as cholesterol be reduced in the diet by more than half now common on American tables and that polyunsaturated fats be substituted for saturated fats as much as possible. Some researchers are convinced that the free radicals caused by the easily oxidized unsaturated fats constantly irritate the artery wall. This is logical when you think how irritating to the stomach fat-fried foods are; the fried fat has combined with oxygen—it has oxidized. This irritating effect of free radicals derived from unsaturated fats is also believed to be responsible for high blood pressure based on its considered effects on the arteries.

Furthermore, the oxidation of polyunsaturated fats depletes the body of its natural antioxidant, vitamin E. Vitamin E is vital to the health of muscles, including the heart, and to blood vessels.

The connection between saturated fats and free radicals, as far as the American Heart Association is concerned, has no credence.

However, the American Medical Association and the American Academy of Sciences differ from the American Heart Association in that they recommend a diet low in saturated fats for the population only at risk—persons, usually young males, who have a high cholesterol at present or who have a family history of cardiovascular disease.

Cancer as well as heart trouble has also been related to the polyunsaturated diet. In experiments with mice, for instance, breast cancer increased as the amount of unsaturated fat in the diet increased. Men in a California veterans hospital kept on a polyunsaturated fat diet developed cancer at a higher rate than those on saturated fat diets.

In Iceland and Japan where large amounts of unsaturated fats are consumed, there is a high incidence of stomach cancer. Similarly, in Sweden and in other countries with a high consumption of fish, which is low in saturated fats, the death rate from gastric cancer of white males in the fifty-five- to sixty-four-year age group is two to three times as high as that for the comparable population in the United States.

Jim Breeling, secretary of the American Medical Association's Food and Nutrition Council said that at this point no one can say whether there is or is not a correlation between unsaturated fats and cancer.

"The work at the California veterans hospital which first suggested the association between unsaturated fats and cancer is being reexamined and it looks as if the correlation is not as strong as previously believed."

However, if oxidized fat and the free radicals it produces are harmful, then what can we do to neutralize them? The answer, a number of researchers feel, is to add an antioxidant to our food.

Two such antioxidants were tested in mice. They were BHT (butylated hydroxytoluene, a common food preservative) and 2-MEA (2-mercaptoethylamine hydrochloride). When added to the diet, they increased the life-span of mice as much as 50 percent.

Larger amounts of antioxidants in our diet may possibly add five to ten years to our lives, and the younger we start the diet, the greater the benefit. However, even if we are elderly, we would achieve significant gains.

Where can we get a safe, widely available, inexpensive antioxidant to add to our food? Without waiting for further scientific proof, thousands of Americans are already gulping one—vitamin E, nature's own antioxidant.

Vitamin E is used in commercial products to keep fats and oils from going rancid, the very process thought to make us age.

The vitamin is controversial, to say the least. Since its discovery in 1922 by two Americans seeking a fertility substance, scientists have attempted to link it to a deficiency disease such as beriberi (lack of vitamin B) or scurvy (lack of vitamin C).

In 1952, for the first time in humans, vitamin E was linked to an illness: a deficiency caused blood problems in premature infants. In 1968 the National Research Council of the National Academy of Sciences set the minimum daily adult requirement for the first time at thirty international units. Government surveys have shown that we are getting about fifteen to seventeen international units in our diet.

Claims for the vitamin range from improved potency and athletic prowess to beautiful skin and a healthy heart.

Vitamin E's link to aging is through a hereditary disease, cystic fibrosis, which usually affects the pancreas, respiratory system, and sweat glands. In 1956 at Johns Hopkins an infant suffering from cystic fibrosis was discovered to have localized muscle lesions similar to those found in E-deficient animals. This led researchers at Columbia University to review the autopsy findings of 151 cases of cystic fibrosis. The lesions, brown deposits, often heavy, were found in the intestinal tract and other tissues of every child who died from the disease over the age of two. Later, an accumulation of the brown deposits, often called ceroids, was found in the central nervous system of six other victims who died of the disease.

The brown deposits seen in cystic fibrosis and vitamin E-deficient conditions in both animals and humans were found as far back as 1894 in the elderly. Even then the nerve cells of the unborn child contained no pigment but the cells of senile humans were largely clogged with it.

The brown deposits of cystic fibrosis are apparently identical to age pigments and the brown pigments found to result from oxidized fat.

Dr. Aloys Tappel, at the University of California at Davis, has been attempting to block aging with vitamin E. He believes that the destruction of fat by oxygen in living humans is the basic cause of the aging of the cell. He believes that ceroid or age pigments are the results of oxidized fat.

This reaction, he claims, is almost completely suppressed by biological antioxidants.

Vitamin E is the only well-known antioxidant that occurs naturally in the membrane of the cell.

Humans, of course, need oxygen to live. But too much of it—hyperoxia—certainly can be harmful. The blindness that occurred in premature infants kept in 100 percent oxygen-filled incubators was proof of this. Volunteers in space capsule research also showed ill effects in their blood from too much oxygen and astronauts during the early Gemini orbital flights also had this blood problem. Vitamin E was given to astronauts prophylactically on other space flights and patients now entering hyperbaric oxygen chambers for treatment of conditions that respond to oxygen under pressure now receive the vitamin prior to entrance.

Vitamin E is also being used to treat and to prevent hardening of the arteries, to protect the heart, and to treat other blood vessel diseases, although such treatments are not accepted by all.

Should we take vitamin E?

The Food and Drug Administration and the American Medical Association claim that it is nontoxic and therefore cannot hurt us; that patients have taken as much as 800 international units a day without ill effect. However, there is some question about high doses being bad for patients with heart failure.

Although the benefits of vitamin E are still controversial, doctors seem to agree that 100 to 400 I.U.s of vitamin E per day won't hurt and may help.

What else in our diet may affect how we age?

Trace elements, so called because at one time they were too small to measure accurately, profoundly affect our health. These micronutrients that move through countless cycles in the environment are in what we eat, drink, breathe, and absorb.

There is still no absolute agreement about which ones

we should have in our diet. Only iron and iodine have official
dietary allowances set by the Food and Nutrition Board of
the National Academy of Sciences.

However, all trace elements are potentially poisonous.
Some are more toxic than others, such as mercury, lead,
arsenic, iodine, beryllium, fluorine, nickel, vanadium, and
cadmium.

A deficiency of some trace elements can, it has been
proven, be harmful to man. These trace elements, in addition
to iron and iodine, include calcium, phosphorus, sodium,
potassium, chlorine, magnesium, copper, zinc, manganese, and
vanadium.

A nutritional deficiency in zinc, for instance, can produce
severe growth retardation, roughened skin, general lethargy,
and a lack of sexual development. It can also affect wound
healing, esepcially in older people.

Nickel has been found to be present in elevated concentrations after a heart attack. This new observation has led researchers to believe that perhaps, in some unknown way,
nickel is vital to human nutrition.

Chromium has unexpected benefits. A frequent problem of
old age is the body's failure to utilize carbohydrates efficiently.
In one study over half the elderly people examined had impaired sugar tolerance, some severe, although not enough to
classify them as diabetics. When they were given supplementary chromium, they handled the sugar normally.

The daily body losses of calcium in the normal adult are
usually about 270 to 370 milligrams per day. Calcium enters
the body through the diet. The National Research Council
recommended daily allowance of calcium is 800 milligrams
for males and females aged eighteen to seventy-five. A glass
of milk per day accompanied by an average amount of cheese,
green vegetables, and bread only provides about 400 milligrams. Thus, a person who had an average or a low consumption of calcium throughout adult life theoretically could have
a serious loss of calcium from the bones in later life. This in
turn could lead to fragile bones—osteoporosis. Gerontologists
emphasize that osteoporosis, which affects so many elderly,

is not a natural part of aging. It is an abnormal condition. Some even claim that tooth loss in later years is not due to decay or plaque but to insufficient calcium.

Until recently, nothing much could be done about fragile bones in old age except cautioning such victims to step carefully. Then it was discovered that adding sodium fluoride to the diet stimulates formation of new bone, and doctors began almost immediately treating osteoporosis victims. But the new bone, it was discovered, was often poorly mineralized and was frequently reabsorbed.

Then, researchers found that by adding calcium and vitamin D along with the fluoride, the bones reformed into youthful strength. In the studies performed at the Mayo Clinic in Rochester, Minnesota, it was determined that dosages had to be balanced carefully. The patients were given 50 milligrams of sodium fluoride; the administration of 45 milligrams did not consistently increase bone formation, while doses of 60 milligrams or more produced abnormal bone. Patients also received two weekly vitamin D supplements of 50,000 units along with 600 milligrams or more of calcium daily.

Milk, of course, is a good source of calcium but so is water. The hardness of water is primarily due to its content of calcium and magnesium. A number of studies have found that the harder the water in an area, the lower the incidence of hardening of the arteries and arteriosclerotic heart disease.

Experimental studies have also shown that blood cholesterol levels as well as hardening the arteries are reduced by calcium and magnesium (whose ions form insoluble soaps with fatty acids in the gut), reducing the amount of free fats in the blood. So if you have naturally hard water, don't soften it.

Another trace metal, vanadium, has been found experimentally to increase, not decrease blood cholesterol.

Still another trace metal, cadmium, has been linked to high blood pressure. Some eminent researchers even go so far as to say that a large percentage of the high blood pressure in this country is due to cadmium in soft water. The metal is leached from pipes supplying soft water. Once in the body, it competes with zinc, replacing it in metabolic activities related to the use of fat. People with atherosclerosis have been found to be deficient in zinc, and it is known that zinc has an affinity for blood vessels. Therefore, cadmium may be a key factor in hardening of the arteries as well as high blood pressure.

How soon we die has always been linked with our diet—in the early days, perhaps because man did not get enough to eat; today, because he may get too much to eat, at least in many Western countries.

The fact is that a man who weighs 154 pounds at the age of thirty and maintains constant exercise over the next thirty years but does not reduce caloric intake will weigh over two hundred pounds by the time he reaches age sixty.

This correlation of decreased caloric requirements with age was developed from an analysis of thirty years of medical records at the Mayo Clinic. The study was originally undertaken to test the theory that fat people used fewer calories for body metabolism than normal, and therefore remained overweight. But, surprisingly, it was found that the basal metabolism rate was normal even in grossly obese persons, even when they performed exercise.

In twenty-two individuals in the study, twelve females and ten males, whose weight had been normal at age thirty, the mean body weight gradually increased until by age forty-two it entered the overweight classification and remained there for the next twenty years.

The basal metabolism did decline as the subjects aged. Because of this, even if the men exercised constantly, they would still have had to decrease their caloric intake by almost 11 percent to keep their weight normal. The women would have had to reduce it by 5 percent over the remaining twenty years to keep their weight normal.

But since most people do not exercise very much, caloric intake probably would have to be cut even more in the average population.

Follow this daily food guide to maintain normal weight throughout life:

	Child	Preteen and Teen	Adult	Aging Adult
Milk or milk products (cups)	2–3	3–4 or more	2 or more	2 or more
Meat, fish, poultry, eggs (average serving)	1–2	3 or more	2 or more	2 or more
Green and yellow vegetables (average serving)	1–2	2	2	1
Citrus fruits and tomatoes (average serving)	1	1–2	1	1–2
Potatoes, other fruits and vegetables (average serving)	1	1	1	0–1
Bread, flour and cereal (average serving)	3–4	4 or more	3–4	2–3
Butter or margarine (tablespoons)	2	2–4	2–3	1–2

Highly recommended: 3 to 5 cups of fluid per day
Reprinted with permission of the American Medical Association

Desirable Adult Weight for Height

	Height (without shoes) Inches	*Weight (without clothing) Pounds*
Men:		
	64	122–144
	66	130–154
	68	137–165
	70	145–173
	72	152–182
	74	160–190
Women:		
	60	100–118
	62	106–124
	64	112–132
	66	119–139
	68	126–146
	70	133–155

CALORIE ALLOWANCES FOR ADULTS
OF AVERAGE PHYSICAL ACTIVITY

	Desirable weight Pounds	Calorie allowance		
		25 years	45 years	65 years
Men:				
	110	2,300	2,050	1,750
	120	2,400	2,200	1,850
	130	2,550	2,300	1,950
	140	2,700	2,450	2,050
	150	2,850	2,550	2,150
	160	3,000	2,700	2,250
	170	3,100	2,800	2,350
	180	3,250	2,950	2,450
	190	3,400	3,050	2,600
Women:				
	90	1,600	1,500	1,250
	100	1,750	1,600	1,350
	110	1,900	1,700	1,450
	120	2,000	1,800	1,500
	130	2,100	1,900	1,600
	140	2,250	2,050	1,700
	150	2,350	2,150	1,800
	160	2,500	2,250	1,900

Reprinted with permission of the American Medical Association

How much should you weigh? Generally, the weight that is desirable for you in your mid-twenties is the weight you should maintain throughout life. Body size, of course, influences the amount of energy or the number of calories required from food.

For example, a man twenty-five years old whose activity is average and whose desirable weight is 150 pounds, needs 2,850 calories a day to maintain that weight. One whose desirable weight is 180 pounds needs 3,250.

Physical activity is a big factor in determining calorie needs. When a person is very active, the number of calories required may be as much as one-fourth higher than when activity is average.

Age also affects calorie needs. A woman of average activity who weighs 130 pounds requires 2,100 calories a day when she is twenty-five years old, 1,900 when she reaches forty-five, and only 1,600 calories at sixty-five years.

Dieting is really very simple. To lose a pound of body fat, you must have 3,500 fewer calories in the diet than the body uses.

If you want to lose one pound a week, your food should provide an average of five hundred calories a day fewer than are required to maintain weight (seven days times five hundred calories). For example, if you maintain weight on 2,300 calories daily, this works out to 1,800 calories a day for a reducing diet. If you have been gaining weight on the amount of food you customarily eat, you will need to cut down by more than five hundred calories a day.

Therefore, to retard aging right now, we should eat a balanced diet and stay away from fad diets. We should forgo softening our drinking water supply if we live in a hard water area. Vitamin E should be used if we're convinced it helps; the psychological lift alone may be worth the price, even if it proves to be limited in its ability to slow the aging process. We shouldn't overfeed our children. We should support university and government researchers studying nutrition and aging, keeping in mind that better understanding of our diet offers the greatest potential for mass control of aging.

Chapter 8

Exercise Can Retard Aging

HUMAN MUSCLE IS AGING earlier today than ever before because, from winking an eye to lifting a carton, increasingly, we are taking those bundles of fibers for granted. And yet, just the coordination of muscles required to get out of bed and walk across a room dwarfs in complexity the most complicated of man-made computers. The workings of the muscles are so complex that science hasn't yet figured it all out.

Muscle makes up 40 percent of our total body weight. There are two main types—voluntary and involuntary.

The voluntary muscles, sometimes called skeletal muscles, will in a healthy person shorten or contract upon command. They are used to walk, run, turn, lift, carry, and so on. Their function is the movement and support of various portions of the skeleton. Each of the about 620 voluntary muscles has its own name, nerve supply, function, and point of origin. All are called striated muscles because each, with its millions of cells, has a striated or crossbanded appearance under the microscope.

However, there is an exception—the heart muscle. Although under the microscope it is striated, we can't start it or stop it at will. It is called an *involuntary* striated muscle.

Not under our voluntary control are smooth, or non-striated, muscles that make up the muscular layers of the intestines, blood vessels, and bladder. But we can easily affect their behavior by certain actions, emotions, and drugs. Examples are eating something that upsets the stomach, anger that might raise blood pressure, or a dose of medicine to calm the intestines. In Eastern culture, particularly Indian, success in control of involuntary muscles through mind power is well documented. The practice is not widely used in the West, with the exception of relatively new research with victims of high blood pressure controlling their hypertension by mental concentration. This also extends to other anatomical functions, and the field is called bio-feedback.

Muscles play a critical role in everything we do from birth to death. They propel us into the world in the first place and keep us moving. They provide nearly all our internal heat. They push food along our digestive tract, draw air into our lungs, expel it, and make it possible for us to have sexual intercourse, and even squeeze tears from our lacrimal glands when we cry.

Life ends when our heart muscle falters and fails after beating approximately 36 million times a year or 2½ billion times in seventy years.

We frequently use the phrase "muscles of iron," yet the contractile element of the muscle is only a soft jelly. How this jelly causes a muscle to contract and lift as much as ten thousand times its own weight is not completely understood.

Our muscular strength that increases throughout childhood and adolescence usually reaches its maximum in early adulthood—earlier in women than in men. How soon thereafter the decline in muscular strength begins depends upon how well we use our own "miracle fibers."

Unfortunately, the ordinary tasks of daily living no longer provide enough vigorous exercise to develop and maintain good muscle tone or cardiovascular and respiratory fitness. In homes, factories, and farms, machines supply the muscle power for most jobs. Mechanization has virtually eliminated the necessity of walking and climbing stairs. Those among us with supposedly the strongest muscles, adult men, spend 25 percent of their leisure time watching television. Many children, who should be exercising and developing their muscles, are driven back and forth to school and then sit in captive idleness before the TV set twenty-one hours a week. And they don't even have to get up to change the channels, thanks to remote control. If some of us do go out for sports, often it is in a golf cart or snowmobile.

This growing disuse of our muscles is increasingly diminishing our entire mental and physical well-being. Many of the so-called infirmities of age such as tottering gait, shaking hands, and stiff joints stem directly from lack of exercise. And such deficits are occuring at a younger age. In recent United States army studies of physical fitness, for instance, some soldiers between the ages of thirty-six and thirty-nine outperformed nineteen- to twenty-one-year-olds. The older men did better in three out of fifteen tests of running, handgripping, and push-ups.

Civilian researchers found the same thing. Young men twenty to thirty years old tended to be in poorer physical condition than thirty- to forty- and forty- to fifty-year-olds.

A common fitness problem now being found among young people is poor posture. Girls seem to thrust their heads forward and round their shoulders, a probable result, according to some researchers, of too much television watching.

Boys, who take part in more active games and carry and lift more than girls, escape this deformity until they get older and less active. But both sexes exhibit the "stance of old age" much sooner than ever before.

And most of us completely give up exercise after we leave school. We give up athletics and use only a small portion of our muscle power.

Exercise not only keeps us looking good, it keeps us feeling good. Co-ed freshmen in Kansas who were considered physically fit had fewer of the common complaints known to most college girls—menstrual discomfort, digestive disorders, backache, fatigue, colds, and allergies.

Extreme lack of movement can quickly start deterioration. A University of Minnesota study showed that total inactivity of muscle caused a loss of strength of approximately 3 percent per day, or 21 percent in a single week. Three healthy men restricted to bed rest for thirty-six weeks experienced a bone strength decrease of from 25 to 45 percent. The greatest loss was in the weight-bearing bones.

Neuromuscular, heart, respiratory, urinary, and skeletal and nervous systems all deteriorate rapidly during prolonged bed rest.

Nevertheless, muscle is the only organ of the body that is easy to rejuvenate. With conditioning exercises, we can have stronger and "younger" muscles at fifty-five years than we had at fifteen years. And there is a great deal of scientific evidence that exercise not only keeps us younger, it greatly prolong our lives.

Physical exertion protects the heart, stimulates digestion, and improves bowel function, making laxatives unnecessary. It helps control obesity and improves posture by toning supporting muscles and it increases brainpower.

In a two-year study of 300,000 men over the age of forty-five, those who never exercised at all had death rates four to five times higher than their associates who consistently exercised a great deal.

British streetcar conductors were compared with streetcar drivers. The drivers, who sat down all day, suffered from more heart trouble than the conductors, who walked around all day.

San Francisco longshoremen tested over twenty years show sedentary longshoremen to have a death rate from coronary heart disease 27 percent higher than those who handled cargo.

Residents of Southern Ireland are known to have one of the longest average life-spans in the world—despite a diet high in milk and beef products containing cholesterol. They live an average of ten years longer than their compatriots because they do hand and arm work such as gardening, woodcutting, and milking cows.

The same beneficial hand and arm work is evidently one reason symphony conductors live so long—Leopold Stokowski (ninety-one), cellist-conductor Pablo Casals (ninety-six), and Otto Klemperer (eighty-eight). Such musicians start their hand-arm exercises early in life and continue every day. (Of course, one cannot discount their love of their work as a factor in longevity.)

The benefits of such hand and arm exercises are available. One can lead an imaginary orchestra while listening to the radio for five minutes every day, or do the more formal exercise of placing the hands at the sides and then swinging them up to meet above the head any number of times, every day, increasing the count as the effort becomes easier.

Mopping the floor or rolling dough can give a similar benefit. One cardiologist believes that housework is the reason women live longer than men and not the difference in hormones or stress. Women exercise when doing housework. The fact that a woman's heart attack rate goes up after menopause does not weaken the theory. That's about the time a woman's family leaves the house, leaving her with fewer physical household chores.

How much exercise we need is still controversial. Logically, if exercise is so beneficial, then athletes should live longer. More and more data is being accumulated to prove that if athletes continue physical activity after their athletic careers end, they do lead healthier, longer lives.

In a classic study of Oxford University crew racers covering 1829 to 1869, their longevity was only slightly greater than that of the average population. However, last year's study of Harvard oarsmen reported a significant advantage: on the average, the Crimson rowers lived to sixty-seven years, six years longer than their nonrowing classmates.

Why should exercising muscles strengthen them, even at an advanced age? The answer may be in creatine, a chemical contained in muscle and believed to be the promoter of muscle growth. Specifically, this agent is essential to muscle contraction but it also appears to act as a "messenger" to stimulate muscle cells to produce more myosin, a muscle-building protein also vital to contraction. In other words, weight lifters may be developing such big muscles because, by lifting weights and contracting their muscles, they are releasing creatine, which in turn stimulates myosin to build more muscle.

The reverse is also possible. Certain cases of muscle atrophy may be arising where a defect in the muscle cell membrane, or envelope, allows the creatine to leak away.

Measuring the differences in creatine and other muscle chemicals and the actual strength of the muscle between the young and the old cannot be done in a resting state. The big variations occur during physiologic stress such as exercise.

Physical exercise reflects the combined capacity of the different organ systems of the body working together. The ability to do work depends on the strength of the muscles, the coordination of movement by the nervous system, the effectiveness of the heart in propelling blood from the lungs to the working muscles, the rate at which air moves in and out of the lungs, the rate of oxygen fed to the blood, the response of the kidneys in removing excess waste materials from the blood, the synchronization of metabolic processes by the endocrine glands, and, finally, the ability of the blood to maintain a chemical balance in the body.

In order to determine the causes of the decline in overall capacity, it is necessary to assess the effects of aging on each of these organ systems.

With a device that measures the strength of the hand, researchers are isolating one aspect of muscle function. Volunteers are asked to squeeze a hand-measuring device as hard as they can.

The average drop in hand strength is from forty-four kilograms at age thirty-five to twenty-three kilograms at age ninety. Also, although the dominant hand is stronger at all ages over the years, it loses more strength than the subordinate hand does. How hard a hand can grip an instrument for one minute drops from twenty-eight kilograms at age twenty to twenty kilograms at age seventy-five.

What does this mean?

The nerve fibers that connect directly with the muscles show little decline in function. The speed of nerve impulses along single nerve fibers in elderly people is only 10 to 15 percent less than it is in young people. Simple nerve functions involving only a few connections in the spinal cord also remain virtually unimpaired.

However, aging takes its toll in the brain and spinal cord where complex connections are made. We have covered some of these areas in the chapter on the brain, but much still remains to be known.

Because muscles engaged in sustained exercise require extra oxygen, and other nutrients, and produce more waste to be carried away, the heart must work harder. It has to move more blood through the system. Therefore, during exercise, the heart pumps more blood at each stroke, and at a faster rate and higher pressure. Although the resting blood pressure in healthy individuals increases only slightly with age (and we have seen the benefit of that increase in the chapter on the brain) a given amount of exercise will raise the heart and blood pressure in old people more than it will in the young. And when subjects exert themselves to the maximum, the heart of the older person cannot achieve as great an increase in rate as that of the younger person. However, by inducing the extra stress on the heart through regular exercise, many physicians contend that the body becomes "trained" to handle stress and to preserve function.

No one, young or old, should start vigorous exercise without any preceding warm-up activity. In a UCLA School of Medicine study, thirty-one of forty-four healthy firemen developed momentous abnormalities in their electrocardiograms (ECGs) after abruptly starting a strenuous running exercise. When they went through a prior warm-up exercise, however, the abnormality did not show up. The findings may account for some heart attacks suffered by people with normal coronary arteries.

Ordinarily, heart attacks occur in people who have fat-clogged arteries—those leading to the heart. Such obstruction, however, is not always found. But, in certain persons, sudden physical activity could cause such a blood shortage, even if only momentary, resulting in a heart attack.

Skipped or premature ventricular heartbeats have also been found to herald the arrival of fatal disturbances in heart rhythm. Often it is the immediate cause of death following a heart attack. In ventricular fibrillation, the heart fails to pump blood because of erratic, uncoordinated beating of the main chamber.

Exercise can bring on such skipped beats but it also can prevent them. Research and studies have demonstrated this. YMCAs around the country now offer physical exercise programs to counteract the effects of heart disease, high blood pressure, high cholesterol, and overweight. At one Manhattan YMCA, participants, all heart attack victims, are examined by a physician before entering the program and periodically throughout. Results of the exercise are encouraging, considering that the national average for recurrence of heart attacks is five per one hundred men per year. In the Y postcardiac group, only one repeat heart attack occurred in a five-year period, and that man is still active in the program.

To determine exactly how exercise benefits the heart, University of Pittsburgh researchers isolated the hearts of exercised rats and sedentary rats. The hearts of the more active rodents were stronger and pumped better than those of the less active ones. The better heart performance was attributed mainly to the coronary blood vessel's greater ability to deliver oxygen and nutrients to the heart muscle.

A step further in the Pittsburgh researcher's quest for answers revealed that physical conditioning alters the chemistry of the heart. The exercised rats' hearts had more of the active protein enzyme, adenosine triphosphatase (ATPase). ATPase sets off the fuel, adenosine triphosphate (ATP), which is necessary for heart muscle contraction. With more of this chemical available, the heart muscle is presumably able to pump with greater force.

But not only the heart muscle benefits from physical exertion. The heart, although the most important factor, of course, is not the sole supporter of the circulation. The elasticity of the aorta and other great arteries is of importance in maintaining an even flow of blood. And the vasomotor function of the smaller vessels is vital for the selective distribution of the blood to the organs as needed. There are the peripheral veins, with their valves, that act as local pumps for the return of blood to the heart muscles. The better the tone of the muscles, the better is this support to the heart afforded by the veins. The peripheral veins help prevent varicose veins and blood clots caused by poor circulation.

Any exercise will also strengthen the diaphragm, the muscle used in breathing. Also, the deepening of respiration that comes with exercise aids in keeping the lungs in good condition.

Long walks, golfing, cycling, or tennis strengthen the leg muscles. Woodcutting, gardening, fishing, or housework make the arm muscles stronger.

But perhaps the most important benefit of exercise is its retarding effect on the process of atherosclerosis, clogging of the arteries with fat. Muscular metabolism, especially that derived from the vigorous use of the leg muscles during walking, acts to prevent hardening and clogging of the arteries by a means not yet clearly understood.

In experiments with rats, the elderly subjected to exercise-training for three weeks had fewer fat abnormalities associated with age than before they began to exercise.

But does exercise do as much for humans?

In a group of Jersey City men between twenty-seven and fifty-four who walked, jogged, and ran during endurance exercises for four-five minutes each day for twenty days, serum cholesterol and other blood fats, as well as body weight, decreased significantly. The forty-five minute exercisers were compared with similar groups who exercised for fifteen and thirty minutes a day for twenty days. Whereas the thirty-minute exercise group had greater reductions of serum cholesterol and skin-fold fat than did the fifteen-minute exercisers, the forty-five-minute group was the only one with a significant reduction in weight. The loss was seven pounds for the forty-five-minute group, three for the thirty-minute, and two for the fifteen-minute.

The blood that pulses at an increased rate through exercise

carries with it more oxygen to the brain. This helps to make one feel more alert. People often fail to realize that keeping the body in good condition also results in greater emotional stability. A dramatic example of this occurred in experiments at Purdue University with two groups of mixed-age men, between thirty and sixty-five years. One group was physically fit while the other was completely out of shape. Tests showed that the physically fit men were more emotionally stable and confident than their unfit counterparts. But, after four months of conditioning the out-of-shape group, the members acquired a better emotional balance and were near the stability level of the highly fit. They increased in self-confidence and became more extroverted.

Exercise is not only good for the heart and mind, it is also good for the bones. All of us should, in the course of our regular day, be on our feet at least two hours. When we do not put weight on our bones, they become susceptible to fracture. This has been proved at a number of research centers. At the University of California Medical School, for instance, it was determined that people who do not stand on their feet for a sufficient time each day have a tendency to keel over when they do stand. Blood collects in their legs; when they rise from a chair or bed, their blood pressure drops and there isn't sufficient blood supply to the brain, so they faint.

But, admittedly, for many people, standing is painful. Next to the common cold and dental decay, probably no human complaint is more prevalent than aching feet. Surveys show that seven out of ten adults suffer from painful feet.

Women especially are prone to foot problems because they bear children. Pregnancy, and childbirth, shifts one's center of gravity and increases the weight. Also, women now stay home less and are unable to rest their feet during the day.

Men also have their foot problems. In the early draft of World War II, thirty-two out of every one hundred rejections were for some type of serious foot ailment. Surveys reveal that one man in ten is absent from work two to seven days a month for the same reason.

The problems with feet start early. About 40 percent of

all children in the United States develop foot ailments by the age of six.

In standing, the foot carries the dead weight of the body. In average walking, it is jolted with a total foot-pound force of several tons a day. A 150-pound man who walks a mile at three feet a step brings down on his feet a total work load for the whole distance of 132 tons.

Not only must feet serve as shock absorbers and supporters, they also function as levers and catapults. They are masterpieces of engineering. Of the human body's 208 bones, 52 are in the feet. There are 66 joints, 200 ligaments, 40 muscles, and millions of muscle fibers and blood vessels. The top of the foot is supplied by the dorsal artery, which is a continuation of the main artery running down the thigh and over the front of the leg. The dorsal artery may be felt if you place your fingers on the top of the foot over the first metatarsal instep. The other main artery of the foot may be felt behind the anklebone on the inner side of the foot. These arteries divide into little arterioles, which in turn divide into even smaller capillaries, supplying the toes with an extremely rich quantity of blood. The veins that return the blood to the upper portions of the body run alongside the arteries. Valves lift the blood up the leg, against gravity. The leg muscles also act as a circulation pump, working to get the blood back to the heart. That is why walking is so important for health.

Many people, especially the aged, give up walking for fun and health because their feet hurt. To test the condition of your feet, take off your shoes and stockings, and stand on a hard surface.

Look at the toes of one foot. Are they the same size and shape as the corresponding toes of the other foot? If they do not match and some are small or deformed, you are undoubtedly experiencing foot trouble.

A closer examination of your feet may reveal corns, bunions, and calluses, usually caused by uneven pressure against your feet. Take a pen and circle every one of these growths. If you have more than three on a foot, it would be advisable to let a specialist in foot care treat you.

Wet your feet and examine the footprints you make on the flat surface. If they leave marks that look like pancakes, you may have poor arches, which can cause you discomfort. Most cases of broken arches can be corrected quickly by proper arch supports worn inside your shoes. But get advice about the support from a doctor, not a shoe clerk.

When standing barefoot, pick up your shoes and examine them. Are the heels run down? Are the inner rims of the heels uneven? Is one heel higher than the other? What about the toes? Are they wide and comfortable or pointed and curled? If your shoes have any of these defects, it may mean you need professional help for your feet.

If you have no condition in your legs that would counter-indicate it such as blood clots, then you can help to keep your feet and body in good shape by the following: Elevate your feet and flex the toes for about one minute, stopping as soon as the foot becomes pale. Then allow your feet to dangle for one minute. Following this, keep your legs in a horizontal position for one minute. Repeat this entire procedure ten times.

Do not stand in one position for long periods because this contributes to stagnation of circulation. Elevate your feet at various times during the day. This helps improve circulation.

For women, alternate your shoes at the office and at home. Constant use of high heels produces foot and leg changes, which contribute a great deal to foot fatigue. If you are going to use high heels, a selection of shoes with varying heel heights will provide a necessary change.

Soak your feet in tepid water after a day's work or a long hike, followed by hot and cold sprays and a good foot powder.

Keeping on your feet and exercising can help ward off arthritis, the chief crippler of old people in America. The bone joints must be kept active. Moving parts are the prime targets of early degeneration. A perfectly functioning joint is least likely to be affected, whereas a joint that operates imperfectly, for whatever reason, is susceptible. Osteoarthritis usually develops in any joint that has been required to take a lot of punishment or abuse, such as a knee or hip joint. The most likely candidates for the disease are the overweight, or those whose joints have been injured in any way. Joints with hidden defects present at birth are also highly susceptible.

Physicians make every effort to keep arthritics moving. Once a hip joint is allowed to become overly stiff and the range of motion becomes limited, the muscles weaken. The more powerful muscles on the other side of the body tend to take over and what may have been a slight favoring of one side can become a twisting of the body.

Mild exercise can keep the musculoskeletal system fully functioning as we age. Even those of us whose life-style limits joint movements to sitting, standing, and lying down can do something. Our daily routine should include several full knee and hip squats, supporting the body if necessary by holding on to a convenient piece of furniture. The market vendors of Southeast Asia, who squat all day, never develop osteoarthritis of the hip.

Common not only to the aged but to almost every age group is back pain. According to many physicians, much of it results from lack of exercise.

The spine, which is shaped like an "S," varies according to age. In the newborn it is straighter than in the adult. When the infant is able to sit upright at about three months of age, the curve in the neck begins to develop. When the child begins to walk, the curve in his lower back starts to form, reaching its final state in early adult life.

In females, the lower back curve is more pronounced than in males but undergoes flattening during pregnancy, the normal curve is restored rapidly after delivery.

To function correctly and to ward off sudden blows, the spinal column is aided by the trunk muscles. This includes not only the back muscles but stomach and hip muscles, which combine to keep the spinal column erect and to protect it.

How can you prevent a backache and an aging back?

By following the advice of doctors specializing in treating bad backs:

- Avoid high heels, narrow-toed shoes, and tight stockings because they interfere with balance and circulation.
- Do not wear tight girdles because they are a hindrance to stomach muscles and impede natural trunk movements.
- Avoid brassieres with narrow shoulder straps.
- Don't wear collars that are too tight or too high. In addition to inducing backaches, they can lead to stiff necks and tension headaches.
- Be sure pajamas or nightgowns are loose fitting.
- Sleep on a firm mattress. The best are stuffed with horsehair, hog's hair, or felt without springs.
- If you have wide shoulders and sleep on your side, have big enough pillows. Avoid foam-rubber pillows. They tend to keep your neck rigid.
- Don't read in an awkward position.
- Never sit in one position for more than a couple of hours.
- In lifting a heavy object, step close and straddle it. Then, using knee, hip, and back joints, lower your body as in a squat, grasp, and lift slowly.
- When getting out of bed, lie on your side, facing close to the edge. Allow your legs to drop off the edge of the bed to the floor. Using the momentum this creates, gently swing the rest of your body straight up and out of bed.

Simple exercises can keep your joints, muscles, and back in good shape and youthful.

In Bed: Raise your head off the pillow and bring it forward to your chest. Then bring your head back to your pillow. Do this several times slowly.

Lying on your back, with your arms at your sides, breathe deeply several times and then open and close your hands until they feel limber. Raise your right arm above your head slowly and then bring it back to position. Raise your left arm above your head slowly and then bring it back to position.

Raise your right leg as high as you can without too much

strain and then lower it back to the bed. Do the same with the left leg.

Raise both legs together just to the point where you feel a little strain in your stomach muscles and then lower them.

Sit up slowly and put one foot over the edge of the bed and then the other.

Sit on the edge of the bed, hands folded behind your head. Rotate the trunk as far as you can until you face fully to one side, then to the other. Now, facing forward, lift both arms over your head and then try to touch the floor. You will have achieved a full range of motion for most of the major joints.

While watching TV: You can exercise to prevent back-aches while sitting down watching television. Take a deep breath and tighten up the big important abdominal muscles. Pull in the sagging belly and count to fifteen. Then exhale. If you do this every time a commercial comes on, you'll have a stronger back and a flatter stomach.

On the stairs: On the bottom step of a flight of stairs, step up first with one leg, then with the other. Step down in the same order and repeat the cycle five times.

At what age should we stop exercising? Cardiologists maintain there is no set age at which a person long accustomed to vigorous exercising should cease. But for some individuals the amount of evercise and the pace may have to be reduced in later decades. However, many lumbermen, gardeners, sailors, laborers, sportsmen, and other such types who have kept up a vigorous program are able to continue their strenuous work well into their eighties.

But whatever one's profession or continued inactivity, it is never too late to start exercising. Even a bad start in life can be overcome. Take seventy-five-year-old full-time researcher Hulda Crooks at Loma Linda University. She had such poor health as a child she did not finish the sixth grade until she was nineteen years old. She received her degree in dietetics from the university in 1943.

Shortly after, Mrs. Crooks completed a week-long

seventy-mile pack trip through the rugged high Sierras of California. She hiked to the top of her favorite peak, 14,496-foot Mount Whitney, the highest mountain in the continental United States. It was her tenth climb in ten years.

To stay in shape, Mrs. Crooks jogs for a mile in eleven minutes every morning. Her jogging began five years ago and was limited to a slow lope across her backyard. After gradually increasing the backyard laps to six, she started running along the street in front of her house. Her nonstop distance increased from a block to a mile within the first year. She also walks a couple of miles a day. A few weeks prior to her pack trip and Whitney climb, she trained by carrying a forty-pound rock-filled pack on her daily walking routes. Mrs. Crooks is unusual and her routine is certainly not for everyone.

The American Medical Association's recommended exercise regime for physical fitness includes regular proper exercise to preserve mental and physical capacities and to significantly delay the aging process; exercise graded according to age, the inclination to activity, and the state of a person's fitness; and exercise done regularly, not sporadically.

How physically fit are you?

Stand on one foot like a stork. Close your eyes and with hands on hips, try to hold this position for fifteen seconds. If you can, your balance is good and you may be in at least fair physical condition.

Lie on your stomach, face down, arms stretched out in front of you. Without bending them, raise the right arm and left leg, then the left arm and right leg. Do not let arms and legs touch the floor. Hold each position for at least one minute. Your back and your endurance are pretty good if you can do it without too much strain.

The following test of physical fitness is used by the President's Council on Physical Fitness to determine the condition of schoolchildren. The test consists of stepping up and down a platform fourteen to twenty inches high thirty times a minute for four minutes. Pulse rates are taken one, two, and three minutes after the exercise. The three, thirty-second pulse counts taken after the exercise are then added and the following formula is used.

199 or more	Poor
171–198	Fair
150–170	Good
133–149	Very good
132 or less	Excellent

Adults can measure their fitness by taking their own pulse. Watching the second hand on a clock, count your pulse beats during a six-second interval, then multiply by ten to give the pulse beats per minutes. A healthy person will usually exhibit a rate of between sixty and eighty beats when seated and about ninety when standing. During light exercise, a rate of around one hundred is normal. If you physician okays it, you can work up to two hundred beats per minute minus your age (if you are forty, this means you can work up to 160) by exercising about ten minutes per day, gradually increasing your effort until you reach that goal. Once you have reached the maximum for your age and physical condition, you can stay in shape by participating in physical activity—housework, walking, formal exercise, etc.—for a minimum of thirty minutes a day.

Any formal exercise program, however, should be preceded by a physical examination. Some apparently healthy persons may have heart or other problems that do not surface until the stress of exercise. The examination in the doctor's office, in addition to the regular blood pressure, respiration, and heart-sound tests, should include basic body actions, both before and after light exercise. A highly important aspect of beginning an exercise program is to start slowly and gradually to approach the desired level of activity.

Exercise should be less than what produces a degree of fatigue incapable of relief by a few minutes' rest. Initially, walking speed should allow one to cover no more than one mile in twenty minutes. Later, the distance can be extended to three miles at the same speed. Then the pace can be increased to three miles in forty-five minutes. Thereafter, most subjects (it's best to check with a doctor first) can progress to jogging or equally strenuous forms of exercise.

Set your own pace, even when exercising with others, and do not try to keep up with the group.

Untoward or unexpected symptoms should bring all activity to a halt immediately. If these symptoms do not subside promptly, a visit to a physician is in order. Warning symptoms might be fatigue accompanied by anxiety, depression, chest pain or presure, headache or dizziness.

The type of exercise is not the critical factor in a reconditioning program. Any exercise that increases the pulse rate, such as walking, bicycling, swimming, or jogging, is beneficial. Pick one that you really enjoy or you will soon give it up.

Chapter 9

The Urge That Never Grows Old

OUR HUMAN NEED TO be loved, touched, and valued never grows old. Fortunately, we are able to fulfill that need throughout our lives—if we are reasonably healthy—through sexual intercourse. There is no specific age barrier beyond which we become incapable of coitus.

Frank Sinatra, Justice William Douglas, and Georgie Jessel are celebrated examples that the fires of romance do not burn low after fifty years. In fact, Charlie Chaplin produced eight living examples that potency is not passé after a certain age. Furthermore, the Russians report a man who fathered a child at 100 years and another from whom healthy sperm was taken at the age of 119 years.

The pioneer sex researcher Alfred Kinsey found that more than 80 percent of the healthy married men and women he questioned were sexually active at age seventy years.

Current sex researchers Dr. William Masters and Dr. Virginia Johnson Masters have found men of eighty-nine and women of seventy-eight still joyfully participating in sexual relations.

Perhaps not always joyfully. Henry Bagley at seventy-three years became the father of triplets, adding to his previous four-marriage progeny of seven children. This does not include his pretriplet four children he gave his wife during their twenty-three years together. He's worried about having more: "We can hardly make ends meet now," referring to his "old age" Social Security and union pensions.

Society overemphasizes sex in youth and middle age. In

old age, it's underemphasized. Sexual intercourse at seventy is considered awkward, ridiculous, or sinful.

Why? Because we live in a youth-oriented society dominated by an insatiable need for newness—resulting in rapid obsolescence that sees no difference between products and people. And we all abet this myopia by trying to look and sound younger with every passing year. Also, there is still a strong, residual underlying feeling that sex without the potential of procreation is unnatural.

With the emphasis on youth and athletic performance and beauty, and the obvious repugnance of society for sexual activity among the aging, it is no wonder that so many people past fifty become impotent or frigid.

Yet, those experts who deal with sexual dysfunction are reporting that young, middle-aged, and old couples share the same sexual problems, including impotency, failure to achieve orgasm, and general incompatibility.

Sexual expression, after all, emanates from the mind and the emotions. Depression about aging, marital troubles, or fears about heart trouble or surgery may all be underlying factors. One problem, which may be magnified among older women, however, is lack of an available partner, although this can occur at any age.

Rarely is there a physical cause for frigidity or impotence. The proof is that Masters and his wife have been able to restore potency in 65 percent of their elderly male patients.

The man is most affected by any decrease in sexual prowess because he has to make a greater physiological preparation for intercourse.

Early male symptoms of the aging process show up during the excitement phase of his sexual response. At fifty years or so, it generally takes the man longer to achieve a full erection than when he was twenty or thirty years. But he is fully capable of achieving that full erection.

However, when a man becomes aware of his slowness, he often panics and believes he is approaching the inevitable decline in potency. He then develops growing fears about his sexual ability and may either avoid sexual contact or find

himself completely incapable of performing during intercourse.

The human penile erection system is a complicated mechanism. It depends upon a fine integration of electrical signals
from the spinal column, normal erectile tissue, and an adequate blood supply to the penis. It is a reflex phenomenon
over which man has little voluntary control. For example, the
sight of a nude female will for the healthy, average male
cause him to have an erection. Yet, it is within the brain that
impotence most often occurs. The location of the particular
brain tissue that affects erection has not, as yet, been definitely
pinpointed. Electrodes have been implanted in the septal region, deep in the center of the human brain. When activated,
the electrodes caused pleasurable sensations and occasionally
penile erection. Conversely, temporal lobe lesions in the brain,
on the side of the head above the ear, have been associated
with loss of erectile ability. But the patient's libido, or sexual
desire, remained normal.

That a cerebral lesion can cause complete impotence
mystifies researchers because electrical signals from the brain
are not absolutely necessary for an erection. Patients with
completely severed spinal cords—cutting off impulses from
brain to penis—continue to have erections. Further research
on the physiologic mechanisms and anatomic pathways that
control participation by the brain in erection success will
help us understand how psychological factors cause impotence.

What do we know about the process of erection?

The actual transformation of the penis from a flaccid to
an erect state is a blood-vessel phenomenon. Blood reaches the
organ from the right and left pudendal arteries in the groin.
These vessels carry blood to the "erectile tissues" of the penis,
the corpora cavernosa—two columns lying side by side—and
the corpus spongiosum, a single column located between
and below the other two. The corpus spongiosum surrounds
the tube that carries urine out of the body. These erectile
tissues are irregular spongelike vascular compartments inter-
spersed between arteries and veins. When the penis is flaccid,

the vascular compartments or spaces contain very little blood and are almost collapsed. When erection occurs, the vascular spaces are transformed into large, distended cavities filled with blood under high pressure.

The distension of the penis with blood during erection is permitted by the relaxing of valvelike structures called "polsters." Polsters contain smooth muscle and are located at the junction of minute arteries and the empty vascular spaces. Under the control of the autonomic nervous system, with fibers running from the spinal cord erection-control centers, the polsters are ordinarily firm and shunt blood away from the erectile tissues into the veins.

When the polsters receive signals for erection, they relax and allow a greatly increased volume of blood to flow into the vascular spaces of the erectile tissue. The rate of arterial flow is temporarily greater than the rate of venous outflow, thus causing the characteristic increase in penile volume during erection. A steady state is eventually reached, where the rates of inflow and outflow are equal and the penis ceases to enlarge but remains rigid.

If the psychologic or reflex stimulus is not maintained for sufficient time, detumescence, or a softening of the penis, normally occurs within seconds. It is not known whether this is merely due to a diminution of the blood-vessel dilating impulses that open the polsters or whether there is some active blood-vessel constricting impulses involved.

When ejaculation takes place, erection subsides promptly because of the sympthetic nerve impulses that facilitate the emission of semen; these nerve impulses simultaneously constrict the vessels supplying blood to the erectile tissues of the penis. Persistence of these impulses even after ejaculation might explain the latent period between ejaculation and the ability to have another erection right away.

Before ejaculation occurs, however, the testicles, which swell in size up to 50 percent during sexual excitement, must be elevated. In men over fifty years, the testicles may not be raised as high as in younger men but they must still be physiologically elevated for an orgasm to occur.

As a man ages, there is often an obvious reduction in seminal-fluid volume during orgasm. There may also be a reduced ejaculatory force if ejaculation occurred previously within the past twenty-four to thirty-six hours; also if a long excitement phase immediately preceded intercourse.

There may be an obvious reduction in the frequency with which a man desires or is able to ejaculate. A male who has indulged in intercourse once or twice a week by his middle or late sixties may need ejaculatory release of sexual tension no more than once a week or three times a month.

A wife filled with the usual "young wives' tales," or instructions from a sex manual, may feel she is not fulfilling her husband if he does not ejaculate every time they have intercourse. If she insists that he does, it can lead him to desire less frequent sexual relations or contribute to impotency by stimulating fears about his performance.

On the other hand, his comfort and potency may depend on how successful he was in his conquests in youth. Chronic prostatitis, or inflammation of the prostate gland, occurs in one man out of three over the age of thirty-five years and is be-believed due, in part, to the "unsuccessful wolf syndrome," or sexual excitement without gratification. Unrelieved congestion makes the gland vulnerable to infection. An infected or inflamed prostate causes symptoms of urinary dysfunction, low back pain, testicular aching, and early-morning discharge.

The prostate is a firm, chestnut-shaped body consisting partly of glandular material and partly of muscle. It surrounds the opening of the tube that carries the urine and is connected to the ejaculatory ducts that store sperm made in the testis. The seminal vesicles empty into the prostate where the sperm cells are mixed with the milky fluid manufactured in the prostate and discharged into the urethra and ejaculated through the penis by a series of contractions.

An enlarged prostate is common in men over sixty years. Its symptoms include progressive urinary frequency and urgency, hesitancy, and intermittency of the urinary stream, and blood in the urine. An enlarged prostate can lead to bladder and kidney infections.

The prostate (and the breast) is highly sensitive to hormones. In the normal male at birth the prostate is enlarged, presumably because of elevated testosterone output of the infant's testicles (because of the release of placental hormone from the mother). This enlargement of the prostate disappears within the first few weeks of life and maturation of the gland awaits puberty.

At puberty, the male hormones stimulate the growth of the prostate gland. But also involved in the encouragement is the pituitary hormone, prolactin. It has been shown to increase the male hormone uptake of the prostate gland. Current research about the dual role of the male hormones and prolactin offers hope that many problems with the prostate gland may be prevented.

Prostatitis does not affect the ability to perform sexually but does, in some cases, cause more rapid ejaculation than customary. The removal of the prostate gland by surgery does not have any direct effect on a man's ability to attain and hold an erection. However, no ejaculate occurs at the time of orgasm because the ejaculate is propelled backward into the bladder rather than forward. This can have an adverse psychological effect in some men, but physiologically it does not interfere with the mechanics of sex.

Many male physical problems common to the later years, those mentioned in the chapter on hormones and including hardening of the arteries, muscle weakness, diabetes, and arthritis of the spine, may affect the ability to have and hold an erection. Fortunately, blood-vessel surgery can often restore the blood flow to the penis and consequently potency. Spinal surgery to remove constriction caused by arthritic changes has also restored the ability to have an erection and the treatment of diabetes can, in certain cases, restore potency.

In rare instances a lack of male hormone may cause impotency. Replacement therapy can remedy it. One example of treatment would be a combination methyltestosterone and thyroid medication. But even infants sustain erections, and their supply of male hormone is practically nil. So unless there is a large deficiency of hormone, chances are that it is not causing the problem.

Many men who claim they are impotent will awaken in

the morning with an erection, indicating that there is nothing physically wrong with their erectile system. These men are psychologically impotent. The fear of impotence is far more damaging to a man's ability to perform sexual intercourse than is his physical aging.

There is also a fear of the physical strain of intercourse, which affects many older men but also a few younger men as well. During orgasm, a man's breathing rate and heart rate increase considerably. However, the rapid heart rate is sustained for only ten to fifteen seconds and is still below the increased heart rate caused by walking briskly or getting angry. A man's blood pressure also rises during sexual excitement. Yet, physicians agree that rarely is sexual intercourse physically dangerous, even for those with advanced heart disease. However, they do point out that sex with a spouse is less strenuous than with an extramarital partner since the combination of fear and guilt may make the sex act more strenuous.

Because society associates the manliness of a man with his sexual potency, many aging males have sought aphrodisiacs, or sex stimulants. Historically, these are supposedly the oldest known class of drugs. The first recorded recipes were allegedly found on a Babylonian cuneiform tablet dated around 800 B.C. It read: "If a man's potency comes to an end catch a male partridge. Pluck its wings. Strangle it and flatten it and scatter salt on it. Dry it. Pound it up together with mountain dadanu plant and give it to him to drink in beer and then that man will get potency."

Actually, a safe, effective aphrodisiac has never been proved. Most attempt to irritate the bladder or stimulate the central nervous system. Alcohol and marijuana supposedly, in small doses, temporarily help potency by relaxing inhibitions. There is no proof of this, and impotency is one of the problems faced by alcoholics. The abuse of drugs may be causing irreparable harm to potency. Ingested or injected drugs appear within a day or two in the male reproduction organs and semen. But they are not ejaculated in spermatozoa until approximately two months, when spermatogenesis (the interval to manufacture sperm) is completed.

Alcohol passes rapidly into the seminal plasma but does not seem adversely to affect sperm. The antibiotic tetracycline, however, soon appears in the seminal plasma and is subsequently absorbed by the spermatozoa. Thalidomide, ingested by male rabbits, can be detected in their semen within a few hours. And it remains in the spermatozoa for nearly two weeks.

The tranquilizer chlorpromazine weakens erection and delays ejaculation; and the tranquilizer/blood-pressure-lowering drug reserpine has similar effects.

Drugs capable of blocking the release of hormones from the pituitary gland are suspected of inhibiting sexual functions; anti-ejaculatory effects have also been reported for other drugs, including chlordiazepoxide (Librium) and phenelzine (Nardil).

Although very little can be demonstrated clinically about the adverse effects of drugs on male potency, drug experts are certain that these effects do occur with commonly used medications. Their avoidance could restore potency in some cases.

However, if potency failure is due to irreparable psychological or physical reasons, there is still help, even though it may not be chemical. Electrical stimulation of the heart and urinary bladders with pacemakers keeps these organs functioning. And both bulls and men have been made to ejaculate electrically, so why not a pacemaker for the penis?

A joint effort by Baylor University and University of Minnesota researchers has produced an implantable erector set. A plastic, hydraulic pump system consisting of two columns is implanted in the penis. An inflation bulb is implanted in one testicle and a deflation bulb in the other. The penile erection produced by inflation is satisfactory to both the man and his partner. The device has already been successfully implanted in seven males, the oldest of whom, at this writing, is sixty-five years and the youngest seventeen years.

A number of physicians anticipate penis transplants, but that would require microscopic techniques because of the number and size of the blood vessels feeding into the organ.

The technology of such an operation is in development. And we have only to overcome an unaware public and perhaps the patient's psychological reaction.

In the meantime there are consolations for most older men. Their experience and greater control over ejaculation has made them better lovers than when they were twenty or forty years old, and it is common today to see older men with younger women.

We've already discussed women's psychological problem about sexual ability in later years. But like men, they can function indefinitely if in reasonably good health.

In many primitive societies women look forward eagerly to the menopause as a time when childbearing is over and menstruation taboos are no longer necessary. Indeed, even highly civilized women may look forward to the menopause when premenstrual tensions become a thing of the past; there is no monthly discharge with which to contend and no need for contraception. But, unfortunately, in America, menopause is feared. Some women still believe that sex after the menses cease is unnatural. This attitude intrudes not only on a woman's sex life but strikes at her whole self-image, complicating and distorting her interpersonal relations in marriage.

For some women, however, sexual relations are enjoyed for the first time after menopause because they need no longer fear pregnancy and are free of young children and can indulge themselves at last. This new interest in sex can create its own problems. Men usually are older than their wives. Sexual activity in young males comes early and spontaneously, but full sexual response in females is more likely learned, and it flowers at forty years or older. Once learned, this female response rises gradually in intensity and often is maintained into old age. Responding to the increased or sustained demands of a woman can put a burden on the aging male.

Women of sixty, seventy, or eighty or more can experience orgasm. For some, it may be painful. A young woman may have regular contractions upon reaching a sexual climax. The postmenopausal woman may have uterine musculature contractions spastically for as long as a minute and a half to two minutes during orgasm. This reaction is experienced by the woman as a sudden, severe, lower abdominal pain followed by postcoital discomfort. The cause usually is a lack of female hormone, medically an easily remedied situation.

In postmenopausal years there is frequently a loss of elasticity of the vagina and sometimes a constriction in vaginal length and width. The involuntary expansion of the vagina to sexual stimulation that occurs in the twenty- to thirty-year-old rarely occurs in a woman after sixty years. If it does, it does so at a much slower rate. But this lack of expansion does not often prevent intercourse and, in fact, may make it more pleasurable.

After the menses cease, the mucosal lining of the vagina usually becomes very thin and atrophic. Forceful coital thrusting may actually split the vaginal wall so that local irritation and even bleeding may occur. We've seen that such problems may be greatly relieved by the selective administration of hormones, either orally or topically. But, ironically, many women are reluctant to discuss this sexual problem with their doctors.

Aging may bring about loss of some of the fatty tissue of the external genitalia, with constriction of the vaginal outlet. Localized pain and distension may hamper initial penetration, or thrusting freedom, by the penis during intercourse. Again, administration of hormones, or surgery, may correct the discomfort.

The female breast is worshipped in the United States as a measure of sexual desirability. The bigger and higher, the better. After menopause, the breast may atrophy somewhat, and sag. However, the use of a well-fitting bra throughout adulthood may help to prevent the sagging. Today's braless girls may well be tomorrow's breast-sagging matrons. Continued physical exercise and good posture can also prevent stretching of the muscles that support the breasts.

Atrophy of the breast can be prevented or reduced by supplemental hormones prescribed by a physican.

But the most devastating injury to the breast is breast cancer. It is the most common form of the disease among

American women. Surgery to remove a cancerous breast may be overwhelming, psychologically and sexually, to a woman and to her husband. Its removal easily leads to a woman's sense of loss of femininity and desirability. However, the American Cancer Society has a special program to help women (and husbands) overcome the psychological ramifications of breast removal.

Another operation that may affect a woman's sex life is a hysterectomy—the removal of the uterus.

Contrary to general, misinformed public belief, the uterus has nothing to do with sexual desire, cleanliness, sexual function, or physical attractiveness. As with other problems concerning impotency and frigidity, it's all in the mind.

There are certainly physical causes of sexual malfunction. In addition to those mentioned, we have already seen that a lack of certain hormone stimulators from the pituitary can abolish sexual desire in both males and females. But, like the other physiological causes of sexual dysfunction, medical attention can correct it.

As far as psychological reasons for lack of a good sex life in older years, contrary to popular belief, aging couples do not refrain from sex because of boredom. Sexual dysfunction is generally caused by a lack of response in one partner. Aging persons are known to fear death less than they do rejection by loved ones. Impotency, or frigidity, for the one, therefore, is painful to both partners, and most likely results from problems that can be remedied medically and/or psychologically.

Naturally, the ability to respond sexually does diminish, though slightly, for both male and female as the years go by. Their skin is less sensitive, their blood vessels and muscles are less responsive, and their secretions more spare. But with regular, loving sexual stimulation, the ability to respond will remain indefinitely, a gift that is uniquely human.

Chapter 10

The Environment for Staying Young

WHEN WILLIAM AND HATTIE Andrews observed their seventieth wedding anniversary in Darlington, Wisconsin, recently, Mr. Andrews was asked for an explanation of the couple's longevity. He replied: "What kept me going was I chewed tobacco for the last eighty years. She fought it—and that's what kept her going!"

The contributions of the internal factors—the strengths inherent in the genes, the innate health of the body—to youthfulness and longevity have been described in other chapters. But what about the external factors—where we live, our satisfaction with our work, our happiness in marriage, and our exposure to the emotional and physical stresses of today's environment?

Such aspects profoundly affect our youthfulness and longevity and we certainly have more control over them than we do over our heredity.

Where we choose to live, for instance, may greatly influence how long we live. Epidemiological studies have shown that if we live in the United States, our chances of a long life are less than if we live in the Scandinavian countries or the Netherlands. It's not just heredity either, because those people residing in Scotland have a death rate 20 percent higher than their cousins in England and Wales!

Since 1920, the life expectancy of the middle-aged American male has increased by less than two years. Currently, it is lower than the life expectancy for men in such developing countries as Albania, Costa Rica, and Portugal.

American women may be longer-lived than American men but they do not live as long on the average as women from Scandinavian countries, the Netherlands, or Canada.

Why? No one knows for sure but there are certain factors. Climate may be one. Because of a decreased ability to adapt to change in temperature, most elderly would prefer to live out their days in temperate climes. Yet, studies have shown that native Floridians live no longer than people elsewhere. However, immigrants to Florida do live longer. Researchers attribute this to the self-selection of those who have the gumption and financial means to immigrate to the state.

Actually, the longest-lived people in the United States reside in the cold climates of North Dakota, Alaska, Nebraska, and Minnesota.

The distribution of diseases is regional, too, so one can increase or lower the odds about contracting a specific ailment. For instance, a white male with heart trouble, or prone to it through inheritance, would be statistically wise to avoid living in New York, Rhode Island, or Washington, D.C. Death rates from heart disease in those areas, respectively, are 393.8 per 100,000; 364.3; and 344.4 compared to death rates for men in New Mexico of 191.1; Arkansas, 201.2; and Kentucky, 211.2.

A white female contrasts even greater. Death rates from heart disease for females in New York are 217.4; 176 for New Jersey; and 175.6 for Rhode Island compared to New Mexico's 83.4; Arizona's 87.8; and Nebraska's 89.7.

Of course, where we choose to live influences our exposure to life-shortening, aging pollutants. An increasing number of scientists believe that environmental pollution is even more important than climate as far as mortality is concerned. One reason is that life expectancy was constantly increasing between the early part of this century until 1960. Now life expectancy has begun to decrease.

The fact is that lowering of the death rate between 1900

and 1960 resulted in a large part from improvements in environmental health.

At least three-quarters of the reduction in death rates came essentially through applied public health measures against infectious diseases and infant and maternal mortality. With proper deference to obstetricians, pediatricians, and prenatal health clinics, more infants are saved through milk and uncontaminated food and water than anything else.

Unfortunately, our air, water, and food are not as pure as they once were. James Watson, who won the Nobel Prize for his work in genetics, feels that Americans are very casual about what they do to their genes; they carelessly introduce chemicals into their environment without knowing the long-term effect.

Among the chemicals in the environment that he and other geneticists believe may harm man's genes are drugs, pesticides, food additives, known cancer-producing compounds, crude extracts of water, and atmospheric pollutants.

If current theories about cancer and aging are correct, anything that can cause adverse genetic effects can also contribute to cancer and aging.

It is estimated that 85 percent of human cancers are caused by environmental factors. The long-term contributions of individual pollutants to cancer and. aging are difficult to determine, but by a happy accident experimental evidence has already evolved in the Lobund Laboratory at Notre Dame University.

Dr. Morris Pollard, director of the laboratory, is raising germ-free rats for a number of experimental purposes, including a study of diet and cancer. Because he was running out of space (there were too many rats in the colonies), he just went around picking out the old rats. At autopsy he noticed some strange things. Those old rats were different. They did not have the malignant tumors seen in other rats their age, and they did not seem to be as "old" physiologically as other rats their age.

In most laboratories 50 percent of the rats die between

fifteen and eighteen months. But 100 percent of Dr. Pollard's rats were alive at two years, and still going strong.

It has been shown in previous chapters that such common factors as smoking, stress, air and food pollutants, excess sunlight radiation, and some common viruses contribute to cancer. Dr. Pollard concentrated on air pollutants and was able to induce malignancies in germ-free rats by exposing them to certain known cancer-causing chemicals found in the air. He was also able to induce cancer with certain viruses. However, when rats were kept completely in the germ-free environment, they did not develop malignancies and they remained amazingly young.

Some of the animals developed thymomas (tumors of the thymus) and breast tumors, both of which were benign. These tumors may be the result of an endocrine gland imbalance or a virus inherited from ancestors not kept in germ-free environments. These animals might not develop cancer and age as fast as other animals because they have filtered air and sterile food and, therefore, are not exposed to antigens. They may consequently have a larger immunologic reserve, an unexpended immunologic competence in old age.

This would fit right into the theory described earlier that aging occurs as our supply of immunity from the thymus decreases.

It would, of course, be hard to raise humans in a germ-free environment, although several babies, at this writing, have been living in a sterile atmosphere since birth because of immunological defects. What happens to these babies and to Dr. Pollard's germ-free animals will provide significant information about cancer and aging. In the meantime epidemiological studies are providing further information about the effects of the environment on longevity. In California, for instance, an association has been found between the use of pesticides and an increased death rate—the first hard evidence that pesticides affect human health.

In California, too, riding on a heavily traveled freeway depleted oxygen in the blood of persons suffering from a painful heart disorder, angina pectoris. As a result, they had increased painful spasms. The researchers who performed the experiments warned that such air pollution is not only danger-ous to angina victims but to everyone, and that those who smoke while riding on a crowded freeway compound the danger.

Links between air pollution and a number of other ail-ments have been made. In Providence, Maryland, residents exposed to fumes from a chemical plant that reclaims dis-carded solvents used in dry cleaning, paint, and lacquer indus-tries had suffered in large numbers from pancreatitis. Air pollution in Buffalo was correlated with an increased incidence of cirrhosis of the liver. Studies of lung cancer deaths among white American males in forty-six states showed that men who lived in urban areas had from 1.56 to 2 times the rate of lung cancer compared to those who lived in rural areas. An-other study showed that smokers who lived in air-polluted cities had a lung cancer death rate 123 percent higher than nonsmokers who lived in rural areas.

Studies of New York and Florida residents at autopsy showed that one-half of all the housewives, blue collar work-ers, and white collar workers in urban areas had unsuspected asbestos fibers in their lungs. Asbestos fibers, when inhaled, have definitely been linked to lung cancer. Asbestos is used in a number of products, including ironing-board covers, pot holders, kitchen tiles, brake linings, and soundproofing tiles. It is also thrown into the air at construction sites during the installation of insulation.

Even the common cold and the flu have been associated in several studies with air pollution. The pollutants irritate the respiratory tract and break down the body's natural defenses against respiratory viruses.

And as for aging itself, chicks exposed to simulated smog began laying eggs at an earlier age than unexposed chicks. The researchers concluded that this was evidence of prema-ture aging.

Our homes are not safe from smog and other forms of pollution.

Noise, for instance, is an increasing problem both out

doors and in. The average kitchen has a noise level of 80 decibels—about as much as a busy street corner. The noise level of a modern kitchen is just below that of the cockpit of an old DC-3.

Every time you hear loud noise at close range you lose a little bit of your hearing ability.

Noise may also cause gastrointestinal upsets, altered responses to allergens, migraine headaches, or an exaggeration of preexisting illness. It can cause a rise in blood pressure, hormonal changes, and insomnia. Noise takes its toll in mental and physical stress. It ages us.

If noise is a problem in the kitchen, so is air pollution. As much as two hundred pounds of grease-laden moisture is given off every year in the average kitchen. If you want to see what you have been breathing, take a look at your kitchen fan.

In a government study in Tennessee, 40 percent of the homes and establishments investigated had one or more appliances that were emitting unduly high levels of carbon monoxide. Gas ranges, ovens, gas floor furnaces, and gas space heaters were most often at fault.

Pollution in the home can kill if it is at a high enough level. If it is subtle but prolonged, it can age us.

What can we do about it?

Keep windows and doors closed when there is significant air pollution outside. Reduce the temperature to 65 degrees and, for short periods, turn on the air conditioner and/or electrostatic filter if you have one.

Keep humidity between 50 and 60 percent year round inside the house.

Choose electric or hot water heat rather than forced air if possible.

Vent clothes dryers outdoors. They are a big source of dust.

Consider noise when purchasing or refurnishing a house. Carpets and bookshelves cut noise. Brick homes are usually the most soundproof, whereas concrete slab houses are the noisiest.

Have only authorized or well-recommended repairmen service home appliances.

Do not bring charcoal grills inside unless the house is well ventilated.

Do not mix cleaning preparations. Deadly chlorine or ammonia gases might be released.

Do not let anyone closer than seven feet to color TV. The danger of X-radiation from color TV has been well documented by government surveys.

Do not spray or use any chemical preparation without reading the label.

Do not use paint or any chemical without keeping a window open.

Be careful about inhaling sprays. Before buying any product, read the label or the directions and consider if the convenience is worth the risk.

Watch what you eat. In America, Canada, the British Isles, and Scandinavian countries, cancer of the large bowel is the second most frequent site of cancer. It is ten times more prevalent in those nations than in developing countries. A link between the concentrated, low-residue, refined diets of Americans and other Westerners with the great prevalence of rectal and colon cancer has been reported. In countries where there is a bulky, high residue, unrefined diet, there is a very low incidence of this type of cancer. Groups that migrate from other countries with a low incidence of gastrointestinal cancer approach the same high incidence of such malignancies in the country of adoption. Vitamin A has been found to exert a delaying effect on gastrointestinal cancer. Yet, surveys in Canada and the United States have shown a widespread, unexplained vitamin A deficiency among large portions of the population. Cancer in all animal organs from ingestion of nitrites and nitrates has been reported by Dr. Samuel S. Epstein and William Lijinsky, Ph.D., of the University of Nebraska. These chemicals are found in certain green vegetables and fruits, in the herbicides 2-4 D, in nitrate fertilizers, and in preservatives added to processed meats, fish, and baby foods. Among the other ingested agents suspected of being

carcinogenic are cycad nuts; the fungus ergot; the mold afla-
toxin; the artificial sweetener saccharine; the pesticide DDT;
and the food additive carboxymethyl cellulose, which is
added to ice cream, soft drinks, baby foods, and a number
of other products. On the other hand, the Russians have reported a very low incidence of stomach cancer in persons living in areas where the soil and water are high in magnesium
salts.

Avoid chronic irritations. If we repeatedly place tar on
the skin, a skin cancer will develop but we do not know why.
Gallstones and bladder stones can lead to severe chronic irritations, which in turn may lead to cancer. The germs of infection, such as bacteria, parasites, or other microorganisms,
are probably not cancer-causing agents in themselves but the
infections that they cause are associated with chronic inflammation, which may lead to cancer. Chronically infected scars,
especially burn scars, and chronically infected cervix all have
been found to be prone to develop cancers probably because
of continued inflammation.

Another "aging" pollutant but one a little harder to avoid
is general radiation. Keep down the number of X rays used
for medical diagnosis by informing the doctor of any available recent X rays. The danger level of radiation has been
estimated at anywhere from thirty to eighty rads. In the
average fluoroscopic examination of the esophagus, stomach,
and duodenum, a total of 21.6 rads are given to the skin.

Dr. John Gofman and his associates at the Atomic Energy Commission-supported Lawrence Radiation Laboratory,
Livermore, California, have warned that there will be 104,000
excess deaths annually from cancer, including leukemia, if
everyone in the United States is exposed to the top "allow-
able" dose of 0.17 rad per year from civilian nuclear energy
application. Some of the Japanese data from radiation exposure of children up to nine years showed solid tumor mortality
increased 3.5 to 7 percent per rad.

The fact that the general public is not now being exposed
to the maximum permissible dose does not impress Dr. Gof-

man. The AEC says the general exposure, including medical X ray, is less than 0.001 rad per year.

Experiments have been going on in two huge underground silos since 1967 to determine how much radiation from cosmic rays affects aging. The air-conditioned, concrete silos—each 174 feet deep and 52 feet across—are in the New York State towns of Ausable Forks and Lewis. White rats and fruit flies are kept in the silos to see if, indeed, cosmic radiation causes aging.

In the meantime, not only can we minimize the effect of pollution at home, we can greatly affect aging and mortality by the occupations we choose.

Chemists have a significantly higher incidence of cancer of the lymph glands and the pancreas. Pancreatic cancers are also reported to occur excessively among workers who are exposed to coal gas and metal dust. Lymphomas have been found to be higher than expected among woodworkers, also among physicians specializing in anesthesiology.

Asbestos workers who smoke run ninety-two times the risk of developing lung cancer compared to nonsmoking, non-asbestos workers.

The least favorable longevity record—characterized by mortality rates about double the rates of all men in a Metropolitan Life Insurance study—was for correspondents and journalists. Men of letters as a group registered a mortality rate 30 percent higher than the average, while government officials experienced a mortality rate nearly 20 percent higher.

Physicians and surgeons showed a death rate of 10 percent higher than average, while business executives and lawyers recorded mortality rates close to the average for all men in the study.

Metropolitan Life statisticians have also studied members of Congress, covering from 1861 through 1968. Members of the House of Representatives had a death rate of 3 percent below the average for the population and senators had a 9 percent lower death rate. A similar study among members of the British House of Commons showed lower rates than that of the general population.

Whereas it seems to be the stress in an occupation that takes the toll, some studies show conflicting results. The Metropolitan Life people compared men in *Who's Who* with others in their profession who were not as successful. The *Who's Who* listees between forty-five and sixty-four years of age had a 3 percent lower death rate. The ambition that led the prominent men to succeed was evidently beneficial, rather than harmful.

Yet, a study of 133 male patients between sixty-five and eighty-five years at the Veterans Administration Hospital, Portland, Oregon, had different results. Those 133 patients had no signs of heart disease, which the researchers attributed to the men's moderate eating habits, a nonfamily history of heart disease, regular physical exercise, normal serum cholesterol, and a collective lack of concern with social status.

How much does stress really age us?

Pollution, overcrowding, traffic, competition—all can make life stressful today. But is a woman isolated in her suburban home with a broken washing machine under more stress than a pioneer housewife isolated from her neighbors and worried about attacks from hostile Indians? Is a motorist under any more stress than a farmer whose income depends on the vagaries of the weather, the insect population, and the price controllers in Washington?

According to Dr. Hans Selye, refugees from Hitler were prime examples of aging by stress. Even if the refugees were anatomically normal, their mortality rate was higher than that of others their age, and they were unable to furnish the same quality of work as the normal workman.

Paranoid patients and depressed patients also show the effects of stress on longevity. Paranoid patients, who turn their aggression outward, live longer than depressed patients, who turn theirs inward.

Poverty, too, takes its toll. People living in impoverished areas with insufficient food and poor hygienic conditions have a much shorter life-span, and they look older than people of the same age with higher standards of living.

If we wish to keep young, perhaps we will have to follow Hamlet's advice and "get thee to a nunnery." Studies of nuns show that they age more slowly with respect to gastrointestinal disease. Their rate is only one-third as great as other American women. The nuns also have an almost total absence of squamous cell cancer of the cervix. Nuns keep working well beyond the age of sixty-five years and have a longer life-span than the average woman.

The causes of death among this select and rare controlled group of American women (115,000 nuns) is most important. Close attention is being paid to their mortality and morbidity. The causes of death among American nuns today, it is believed, anticipate those of American women thirty years hence.

An intriguing question is: Will there be change in their causes of death as American nuns return to the secular world as many are now doing?

Attitudes are so important to health and longevity that we can actually postpone our deaths. A decrease in deaths was noted in the months immediately before birthdays, presidential elections, and among Jews preceding the holy day of Atonement. Johns Hopkins researchers attribute the dip to a desire of the patients to witness critical dates.

A recent government study showed that a group who attended church or synagogue lived longer than others in similar circumstances who did not. Could this be another attitudinal effect on aging and on longevity?

How much does environment—the total environment—affect aging and longevity? The only way to really determine this is to study whole populations of long-lived persons.

A Russian gerontologist did just that with the amazingly long-lived people of Dagestan. He came up with the following basic factors responsible for long life in that republic:

Generally favorable climatic and geographic conditions.

Simple, but highly varied diet of milk products, vegetables, and meat.

Observance of several sound rules of hygiene; moderate, systematic labor throughout life; and normal rest.

Certain daily life traditions, including abstinence from sexual excesses, smoking, and alcohol.

A neuromuscular system well adapted to mountainous conditions; hardening of the body beginning with childhood.

Sound distribution of work in the family.

Heredity.

In a community of longer-lived persons in Vilcabamba, Ecuador, there are a number of residents over one hundred years old, and one who has reached 121 years. The villagers (of European rather than Indian extraction) rise at dawn and work in the fields until nightfall, eight thousand feet above sea level.

The high altitude, low-oxygen environment of Dagestan and Vilcabamba fits into the pattern emerging in geronology laboratories around the world. Oxygen ages the organism; low oxygen concentrations help retard aging.

The Vilcabamba villagers eat a diet of an average 1,700 calories a day, including 153 calories of animal fat. Recall that the American diet contains 2,400 to 2,600 calories per day, 450 to 500 of them animal fat. Blood serum levels of cholesterol in the adults of the Ecuador village average 160 to 165, while the typical blood cholesterol of the American fifty-year-old male is 250.

In studies of long-lived and short-lived persons, long survivors scored higher on test of intelligence, adaptation, morale, and mental health in general. In other studies high intelligence, sound financial status, well-maintained health, and intact marriage were equated with the long-lived. Those with less intelligence, less money, broken marriage, and declining health died sooner.

The factor of happy marriage and longevity continually pops up. Out of 4,486 British widowers fifty-five years of age and older, 2.3 percent died during the first six months of bereavement—40 percent above the expected rate for married men of the same age. In the United States married people have death rates lower than the single, widowed, or divorced at every age. Furthermore, divorced white men and women have higher death rates at almost every age than widowed white men and women.

A long-range study at Duke University figured out the criteria that can help predict how long we will live. During the first examination of 268 persons aged sixty to ninety-four years, age, sex, and race were the best predictors of longevity based on actuarial tables.

The next most important factor was physical functioning, based on medical history, physical and neurological symptoms, audiogram (for hearing), chest X ray, electroencephalogram (brain waves), electrocardiogram, and laboratory studies of blood and urine. The most important single factor in this category was the absence of heart and blood vessel disease. One finding, conflicting with many other studies, is that the presence of higher levels of cholesterol is positively related to longevity, whereas obesity, emaciation, and the amount of tobacco are unimportant.

Work satisfaction turned out to be very important. Among men sixty to sixty-nine, it was the single most important predictor of survival, even better than life-expectancy charts and physical functioning.

Among the women in the study, both work satisfaction and performance intelligence are eliminated as significant factors. Physical functioning—their general health—is most important to women, even more than chronological age.

Intelligence scores closely followed longevity; the smarter, the longer-lived.

Of course, no predictors can be completely accurate. Human factors can fool the statisticians. An example was a white male, aged eighty-one, who entered the study at an actuarial life expectancy of another 5.6 years. The man's health was average, but his work satisfaction was the highest possible, and performance intelligence was high. The study predicted the man should live another 9.5 years but he achieved 11.6 years, more than double the conventional actuarial prediction.

Want to live longer?

The Colorado Medical Society offers this much practical advice regarding the external factors.

- Act your physiologic age. If you are not physically equipped for violent exercise, don't try competitive sports and strenuous exertion just because it's fashionable. On the other hand, if you are well endowed physically, don't let yourself go to pot.

- If you go in for vices, don't concentrate on just one of them. Spread it out—in moderation. Moderate drinkers, for example, live longer than heavy drinkers. Gluttony is particularly bad to cultivate if you want to live a long time.

- Learn to live with yourself. Accept your limitations and disabilities—mentally, physically, and economically. The ease with yourself that you will attain will make life more worth living however short or long the years.

- Move more rationally toward your life goals. Avoid extremes and sudden spurts.

- You should have goals. They should be changing ones —changing with the degree of your maturity and your physical condition but always there to give life flavor and usefulness.

- Don't look forward to retirement as a time when you quit. It's the people who disregard this rule who often die shortly after they retire. Plan for retirement. Look forward to it as a point in life at which you give up one thing in order to do another you very much want to do. Educate yourself for retirement. Most people don't know how to retire.

- Taking good care of yourself involves, as a first requisite, the early diagnosis and prompt treatment of disease at any age. You should see your doctor regularly regardless of the number of your birthdays. Don't balk at treatment on the argument that it's not worthwhile because you're too old and only a few years remain anyway. It is worthwhile, and maybe you have a lot more years in store than you think.

Added to these items of advice, of course, are:

- Keep away from pollution as much as possible both within your home and without.

• Don't smoke. Life expectancy of nonsmokers is about six years greater than that of heavy smokers (more than twenty-one cigarettes a day).

• Have periodic checkups. There are many precancerous conditions that when treated never turn into cancer. Among these are benign tumors—leukoplakia (an overgrowth of cells that often take the form of white patches on the lips, tongue, or inner cheek) and keratosis (small scabs or black warts, particularly on the scalp).

• If you are not married, get married. If you are, work on keeping your marriage healthy.

• Keep your mind sharp by learning new things.

Above all, we must enjoy ourselves if we are to make our longer years worthwhile. At a point of balance between caution and indulgence, there is a sensible way that cannot only add years to our lives but life to our years.

Postscript

NOT ONLY WILL WE be able soon to greatly extend life in our lifetime, we will be able to repair defects and to banish pain and suffering—be it diabetes, heart trouble, mental retardation, or whatever.

Millions and millions of ageless aged not incapacitated and ready for the rocking chair will want to continue living life to the fullest. We will come to know one hundred-year marriages, families of at least six generations, and living experiences and knowledge of centuries vintage.

We will be able to maintain a physical and mental condition of twenty-five-year-olds. We will not develop the age-connected diseases that are today overburdening doctors and health-care facilities. And we will be better able to withstand environmental stress.

Plato taught that the purpose of philosophy was to teach men to achieve noble death. How much easier to contemplate when we know that death and disability are no longer inevitably intertwined.

But will we be more creative, less harried, happier? Not unless we become better prepared for the great increase in life-span—much better than we have for the initial extension of life that has already occurred.

It wasn't long ago that retirement at sixty-five just didn't exist. There were family farms and businesses. Family relationships were firm, and being a parent in itself was a form of insurance for old age. Children generally worked with parents, lived in the same neighborhood or house, and as the parents grew older, the roles gradually reversed. The parents did not formally retire but continued to work with a decreasing work load as the children took over more and more of the work burden.

In 1900 two-thirds of the men over sixty-five years were still at work. Today just one-third are. By 1980, unless we make changes now, just a third of the population over fifty-five will be at work; although most companies still set retirement at sixty-five, the trend is to fifty-five. Some companies already have endorsed early retirement with lowered benefits for ten years of service.

As a result, the social and economic problems of the aged —low income, loss of prestige, isolation—are rapidly becoming applicable to younger and younger "old" people. Since 1972, for example, auto workers could retire with full benefits after thirty years of service. But if they take another job, their benefits would be drastically reduced; the "thirty and out" rule will allow a good many of them to retire as early as forty-seven.

Military personnel can retire after twenty or thirty years' service, regardless of age.

On the average, 10 percent of all retirements today are "early." The rate is three times higher for employees with liberalized early retirement benefits than for those without such provision.

Workers, of course, choose early retirement chiefly because of the increased retirement income. Business encourages early retirement to allow for faster advancement of younger employees, who are considered more motivated and productive. Companies feel that early retirement somehow softens the impact of compulsory retirement policies at age sixty-five because there is a "voluntary" element in it. Union leaders like early retirement because it helps ease unemployment among young married workers—who have largely figured among the militant rank and file.

Social scientists foresee a society in which young people will go to school until they are twenty-five, work until fifty-five, and live until eighty-five or more in retirement. Anyone

in his thirties today will probably spend more years in retirement than on the job.

The aged will come upon us fast. The birth rate in the
United States today is already below the replacement level,
and if each couple continues to have only one or two children
and life continues to be extended, the big change will occur
in *style*, not numbers.

Will future retirees be able to maintain themselves for
another fifty years or more? Will younger workers be able to
support the increasing number of retired? Similar problems
exist now with the growing number of persons on welfare
who are being supported by tax monies.

But just money won't solve this problems. Purposeful activity is inherent in the pursuit of happiness. In our civiliza-
tion we judge a person by his work. The money one earns at
that work buys the necessities and luxuries of life. However,
work lends prestige and gains us acceptance by our relatives,
friends, and neighbors, and contributes to our dignity and
concept of self-worth.

We must build a bridge if we are to avoid a nation of many
aged misanthropes. We must open up resources so that millions of healthy elderly who want a useful, interesting role in
our world can have it. We must challenge our dated concepts
of what old people can and cannot do. We must question now
the idea that they cease to expand as individuals and become
rigid and incapable of creative thought—as the stereotype of
the old settler interviewed on his one hundredth birthday: "I
suppose you've seen a lot of changes in Charleston in your
day?" the reporter asked. "Yes, I have," said the centenarian,
"and I want to tell you, young man, I've been against every
darn one of them."

The benefits of early planning provide for the enjoyment
of life. A ship's musician collected curios and art objects
wherever his ship put into port—from Singapore to Mar-
seilles. Now he owns a popular curio shop in mid-Man-
hattan and finds his retirement years "the most exciting" of
his whole life.

Why not multiple careers? Even if companies maintain early retirement, why must new replacements be chronologically young? With a new start and past experience, new employees could be very valuable at fifty, seventy-five, or even one hundred.

Many women today are finding that they can "recycle" themselves. Suffering from the "empty nest syndrome" that occurs when their children have grown and left home, these women are taking jobs, going back to school, and starting new careers. Hofstra University, Barnard College, Rutgers University, and Newark State, among others, have been quick to see the need. They offer retraining programs for women long out of the labor market. But what about the men who wish to start new careers? Or the retired of either sex?

Starting all over again with new training and a new outlook plus years of past experience and maturity can be rewarding both for the older person and for society. As far as being able to learn new things, Chapter 5 describes how much of the so-called mental incapacity in older people today is really the result of depression and lack of stimulation and not age. As we learn more about the aging process, we will be able to protect our intellect into very old age and, if it starts to fail, restore it with chemicals.

The proof that the aged can be excellent workers is already available. A recent survey showed that workers over the age of sixty-five years performed their jobs about equal to and sometimes better than younger workers. In addition, the survey found that older workers are as punctual in the mornings as younger employees, have fewer on-the-job accidents, and are less often absent from work because of illness.

Many companies are already dealing with retirement more successfully than the common practice. They are not forcing a healthy ambitious person who wants to work out of the labor market, making him feel instantly old, useless, and inferior. These forward-looking companies are retraining pre-retirement personnel for new careers or new avocational interests, and many such retirees do not leave the productive force but embark on second and third careers.

Some of the early and traditional retirees are taking low-paying but vitally necessary public service jobs, which younger people with families to support cannot afford. A number of retired businessmen are now using their years of experience to advise younger businessmen with problems. Elderly people are serving as foster grandparents in hospitals, and as teachers' aides. There are those who find satisfaction in donating their services and those that have so many varied or deep personal interests that the days of their retirement fly happily by. One Harvard professor is using his retirement to contemplate. As his grandson describes him: "He is an old gentleman who sits and thinks a lot—and keeps my mother from hitting me."

There are and always have been compensations for aging. Sophocles when asked if he was still the man he was when young said: "Old age has a great sense of calm and freedom. The passions relax their hold, and we are free from the grasp not only of one mad master but of many."

For many of the ageless aged, freed from the demanding pursuit of money, status, and conquests, they will have time for contemplation and creativity. We might even discover new genius in old age. Perhaps a budding da Vinci or a new Mozart. And what if we were able to expand the productive lifetimes of such men? What had Mozart yet to give us? And Einstein? When the still-living world-famous physiologist Fritz Vezar discovered the physical effects of the renal hormones, it was even before those hormones were isolated. When he retired at the age of sixty-five from his position as professor of physiology at the University of Basel, he bought an old house near the university, set up a laboratory, and completely changed his field of research to gerontology. He has linked the changes in connective tissue to cross-linking and has made other contributions in the field. At eighty-five years, he is still going strong: working, traveling everywhere, climbing mountains. When Dr. Nathan Shock, who gave me this account of Dr. Vezar, visited him, Dr. Vezar outwalked him.

Duke University's Ewald Busse said a man named Joe stands out in his mind:

"It is very fascinating. As Joe's capabilities diminish, he moves to another interest. For instance, after his retirement, he became an avid gardener. When he had trouble with his leg, he moved from gardening to running the Rotary Club meetings and setting up political and social round tables. He has many subinterests."

Making the most of our entire life-span is the ultimate goal of the gerontologists. But that goal can be reached only if the ageless aged among us are valued. The Japanese culture has successfully dealt with its elderly through the ages. The baby was independent in a sense because it was allowed to behave almost as it wished. Gradually, independence was discouraged until a low was reached during the prime of life, with the independence curve gradually ascending until after the age of sixty. Thus, in Japan infancy and old age secured maximum freedom and indulgence.

With industrialization, Japan has changed and they do have many of the same problems with the elderly that we do, but what has remained constant is the Japanese elderly's continuing development of the inner self and self-respect. Here, however, aging brings gradual isolation and unproductive idleness.

But as the ranks of the ageless aged increase, along with the technology to extend active life, so will their power. They will be as the onetime youngsters who protested an unpopular war and the irrelevancy of mass education. Human beings will once again, like fine wine, increase in value with aging. They will have the time to learn about the world within and without them. They will know the reality of Robert Browning's "Grow old along with me!/The best is yet to be."

Background Sources

Chapter 1

PAGE

2   Raymond Harris, M.D., Albany Medical College, *Medical Tribune*, September 5, 1968.

2,8   Benjamin Schloss, Ph.D., president, The Foundation for Aging Research, interview, New York City, November 11, 1970.

3   "Ethical Considerations in Longer Life Span," *Geriatric Focus*, October 1, 1969, vol. 8, no. 16.

3   *Journal of the American Medical Association*, September 11, 1967, vol. 201, no. 11, p. 33.

3   "Health Characteristics of the Elderly, " *Metropolitan Life Statistical Bulletin*, August 1968, vol. 49.

3   Social Security Administration, personal communication with author, March 10, 1971.

3,4   Tamara Abarshalin, Information Department, Embassy of the Union of Soviet Socialist Republics, 1706 Eighteenth Street N.W., Washington, D.C. 20009, personal communication with author, April 28, 1971.
Guinness Book of World Records, 9th ed., May 1970.

4   Edward Henderson, M.D., president, The Aging Research Institute, Inc., New York City, interview, January 10, 1971.

4,5   Ewald Busse, M.D., chairman, Department of Psychiatry, Duke University Medical School, interview, January 24, 1971.

4   Nathan Shock, Ph.D., chief, Gerontology Research Center, National Child Health and Human Development Institute, speech presented at the Fifth International Congress of Dietetics, Washington, D.C., September 12, 1969.

4   Barnes Woodhall and S. Jobolon, "Prospects for Further Increases in Average Longevity," *Geriatrics*, 1957, 12: 586–91; R. R. Cohn, "Human Aging and Disease," *Journal of Chronic Diseases*, 1963, 16: 5–12; Alex Comfort, "The Biological Basis for Increasing Longevity," *Medical Opinion and Review*, April 1970, pp. 18–20.

5   Nathan Shock, Ph.D., "Age with a Future," *The Geron-*

tologist, Autumn 1968, **vol. 8, no. 3, part I, p. 148.**

5   *A New Concept of Aging*, American Medical Association's Committee on Aging, Department of Health Care Services, American Medical Association, 535 North Dearborn Street, Chicago, 1966.
Shock, interview with author, Baltimore, March 3, 1971.

Chapter 2

6,7   James Birren, Ph.D., "Research in the Service of Man"—a conference sponsored by the subcommittee on research, Oklahoma City, October 24–27, 1966.

7,13   Edward Henderson, director, Aging Research Institute, New York City, interview, January 10, 1971.

7   *Metropolitan Life Statistical Bulletin*, July 1970, vol. 51.

7   Health Resources Statistics, U.S. Department of Health, Education and Welfare, 1969, p. 131.

7   E. Cuyler Hammond, Sc.D., of the American Cancer Society, "Analysis of the Association Between Cigarette Smoking and Mortality," paper presented at the American Association for the Advancement of Science, December 28, 1971.

7   The Gerontology Research Center, National Institute of Child Health and Development, August 1969.

7   *A New Concept of Aging*, American Medical Association's Committee on Aging, Department of Health Care Services, American Medical Association, 535 North Dearborn Street, Chicago, 1966.

8   Nathan Shock, Ph.D., "The Beginning of Deterioration," in *The Art of Predictive Medicine* by Webster L. Marxer, M.D., and George R. Cowgill, Ph.D., Springfield, Ill.: Charles C. Thomas, p. 1.

8,10,11   A gerontology research section of the National Institutes of Health was established at the Baltimore City Hospitals in July 1940. In 1959, as part of its program, more than six hundred healthy, community-dwelling men, aged twenty to ninety-five years, were enlisted to undergo periodic examinations. The exams included extensive series of biochemical, physiological, medical, and psychological tests to measure individual changes with aging.

9,12 Nathan Shock, Ph.D., interview with author, March 3, 1971, Baltimore.

9 Sir George Pickering, "Degenerative Diseases: Past, Present and Future," presented at "Reflections on Research and the Future of Medicine," symposium cosponsored by Columbia University and Merck Sharp & Dohme Research Laboratories, March 26, 1966.

10,11,12 Ewald Busse, M.D., chairman, Department of Psychiatry, Duke University Medical Center, with a grant from the National Institutes of Health, established an interdisciplinary research project on the relationships of physiological, psychological, and social factors to the process of aging. Some 260 community volunteers over sixty years of age have participated. They undergo comprehensive medical, psychological, psychiatric, and social history evaluations at regular intervals. Sixty-seven percent are white, 33 percent Negro; 41 percent male and 59 percent female.

The Gerontology Research Center, National Institute of Child Health and Development, August 1969.

10 Richard Kronenberg, M.D., et al., "The Effect of Aging on Lung Perfusion," *Annals of Internal Medicine*, March 1972, 76: 413–21.

12 "Blood Pressure Does Not Inevitably Rise with Age," *Medical Tribune*, February 9, 1972, vol. 13, no. 6, p. 1.

Chapter 3

13,14 Messam Fikry, M.D., "The Aging Cell: Aging and Death as Aspects of Growth and Development: Natural Phenomena Controlled by Genetic Factors," *American Geriatrics Society Journal*, November 1969, vol. 17, pp. 1044–54.

14 Howard J. Curtis, "Biological Mechanisms Underlying the Aging Process," *Science*, August 23, 1963, pp. 686–94.

14 *A Full Measure of Life: Support of Aging Research*, a publication of the National Institute of Child Health and Human Development, June 1969.

14,15 Charles Barrows, Jr., Sc.D., interview with author, March 3, 1971, Baltimore.

15 Nathan Shock, Ph.D., "Perspectives of the Aging Process," Psychiatric Research Report 23, American Psychiatric Association, February 1968.

17 Marie-Louise Johnson, Ph.D., *Science Digest*, October 1968, p. 59.

19 Samuel S. Epstein, M.D., of Harvard, Chief of the Laboratories of Environmental Pathology and Carcinogenesis, report presented to the 60th annual meeting of the American Association for Cancer Research, San Francisco, March 23, 1969.

19 Johan Bjorkstein, "Chemistry of Duplication," *Chemical Industries*, 1942, 50:69; Bjorksten, "Cross Linkages in Protein Chemistry," New York, Academic Press, Inc., 1951, vol. 6, pp. 342–81.

20 Ewald Busse, M.D., "Geriatrics Today—An Overview," *American Journal of Psychiatry*, April 10, 1967, 123:1226–33.

21 M. A. Rudzinska and R. K. Poter, "Observations on the Fine Macronucleus of the Tokophrya Infusiorium," *Journal of Biophysics-Biochemistry and Cytology*, 1955, 1:421–28.

21,22 Nathan Shock, Ph.D., "Is an Organism's Life Programmed?" *American Professional Pharmacist*, January 1969, pps. 42–47.

21 Donald G. Carpenter, Ph.D., and James H. Loynd, M.D., "An Integrated Theory of Aging," *Journal of the American Geriatrics Society*, December 1968, vol. 801, pp. 1307–21.

21,22 Hans Selye, Ph.D., *The Stress of Life*, New York, McGraw-Hill, 1956.

22 "Evidence Is Found That Aging Turns Off Protein Synthesis," *Medical Tribune*, October 6, 1971, p. 1.

22 "A Substance Chemically Like Motor Oil Helps Arteries Stay Young and Flexible," special research report issued by the American Heart Association, 44 East 23rd Street, New York, N.Y. 10010, May 10, 1972.

23 Nathan Shock, Ph.D., interview with author, March 3, 1971, Baltimore.

Chapter 4

24 Data from the National Natality and Mortality Surveys. Series

22, Public Health Service Publications, 1970.

24   "American Longevity in 1968," *Metropolitan Life Statistical Bulletin,* August 1970.

24   Data on Natality, Marriage and Divorce, Series 21, U.S. Department of Health, Education and Welfare, 1970.

26,27   James B. Hamilton, Ph.D., personal communication with author, March-April 1971, James B. Hamilton, Ph.D., and Gordon Mestler, "Mortality and Survival: A Comparison of Eunuchs with Intact Men and Women," presented at the American Association of Anatomists, Boston, April 2, 1970.

28,30   Herbert S. Kupperman, M.D., Ivan S. Young, M.D., Julianne L. Imperator, M.D., and Paul Beck, M.D., "Pharmacologic Properties and Clinical Effects of Estrogen in the Human," New York University pamphlet.

28,30,32   Herbert S. Kupperman, M.D., interview with author, March 25, 1971, New York.

29   Kang-Je Ho, M.D., Paceto Manalo-Estrella, M.D., and C. Bruce Taylor, M.D., "Female Sex Hormones," *Archives of Pathology,* August 1970, vol 90.

31,32   Herbert S. Kupperman, M.D., "The Female Climacteric," *Management of the Principal Symptoms of the Menopausal Patient,* February 1969, vol. 1, no. 1.

31   Hector Castellanos, M.D., symposium on the ovary, Temple University, November 15, 1967.

31   "Did an Ovary Transplant Work?" *Medical World News,* March 19, 1971.

32   "Estrogens—Why Harmless as Menopausal Therapy But Hazardous in the Pill?" *Journal of the American Medical Association,* Question and Answer Section, January 18, 1971, vol. 215, no. 3, p. 292.

32   Thomas McGavack, M.D., correspondence with author, April–May 1971, and "The Male Climacterium," *Journal of The American Geriatrics Society,* September 1955, vol. III, no. 9, pp. 639–55.

Robert Morgan, St. Bonaventure University, *Perception and Motor Skills,* February 27, 1968, pp. 595–99.

32,33   W. Donner Denckla, M.D., Department of Physiological Chemistry, Roche Institute of Molecular Biology, Federation of American Societies for Experimental Biology, April 15, 1971, Chicago.

33   "Prolonged Benefits from Calcium Infusions in Osteoporosis," National Institute of Health News Report, September 1, 1970.

35   "The Role of Biological Clocks in Mental and Physical Health," Investigator Curt P. Richter, M.D., prepared by Gay Luce, Behavioral Sciences and Mental Health, National Institutes of Health publication.

36   Julius Axelrod, Ph.D., and R. J. Wurtman, "The Formation, Metabolism and Some Actions of Melatonin, A Pineal Gland Substance," in *Endocrines and the Central Nervous System,* Washington, D.C., 1966.

36   Reuben Andres, M.D., "Aging, Glucose Tolerance and Diabetes—A Proposal," chapter 10, *Endocrines and Aging,* edited by Leo Gitman, M.D., Springfield, Illinois: Charles C. Thomas, 1967.

36   *Medical World News,* February 1, 1971, p. 32.

37,38   Eugene A. Cornelius, M.D., Ph.D., "Induction of Tumors and Autoimmune Changes in Neonatality," presented at the Federation of American Societies for Experimental Biology, Chicago, April 14, 1971.

37,38   "Mature Thymus Transplants May Now Be Clinically Possible," *Journal of American Medical Association,* July 3, 1972, vol. 221, no. 1.

39   Research Association, "A Century of Life," *Medical World News,* June 12, 1970, p. 28.

39   Press reports, January 7, 1971.

39   The National Institute of Health Record, January 19, 1971, vol. XXIII, no. 2, pps. 1–3.

40   Walter Sullivan, "Man Made Molecule to Ease Growing Pains," *The New York Times,* January 10, 1971.

39,40   Nathan Shock, Ph.D., director, NIH Gerontology Research Center, interview with author, March 3, 1971, Baltimore.

39,40   William H. Harris, M.D., Associate Clinical Professor of Medicine, Harvard, paper presented at the American Academy of Orthopedic Surgeons. January 17, 1970. Chicago.

40   Dietrich Bodenstein, Ph.D., "Contributions to the Problem of Regeneration in Insects," *Journal of Experimental Zoology,* June 1955, vol. 129, no. 1, pp. 209–24.

40   **Robert O. Becker, M.D.,** and David Murray, M.D., "The Electrical Control System Regulating Fracture Healing in Amphibians," *Clinical Orthopaedics and Related Research,* Marshall R. Urist, editor, J. B. Lippincott and Co., 1970.

40   "Limb Regrowth Held Possible," Medical News Section, *Journal of the American Medical Association,* June 1, 1970, vol. 212, no. 9, p. 1443.

Chapter 5

42   *Working with Older People: A Guide to Practice,* vol. III, U.S. Department of Health, Education and Welfare, April 1970, p. 36.

42   D. Trembly and J. O'Conner, "Growth and Decline of Natural and Acquired Intellectual Characteristics," *Journal of Gerontology,* 1966, vol. 21, pp. 9–12.

42   "At Age 100, Inventor Champions Sun Power," *National Geographic News Bulletin,* April 14, 1972.

43   L. H. Elam and H. T. Blumenthal, "Aging in the Mentally Retarded," Interdisciplinary Topics of Gerontology, New York: Karger, Basel/Munich, 1970.

43   "Boy 12 Dies of Old Age," United Press International, January 29, 1971.

44,45,46   Ewald Busse, M.D., "Therapeutic Implications of Basic Research with the Aged," The Institute of Pennsylvania Hospital's Strecker Monograph Series, 1967, no. IV.

47   Larry Thompson, Ph.D., and Stuart Wilson, Ph.D., "Electrocortical Reactivity and Learning in the Elderly," *Journal of Gerontology,* January 1966, vol. 21, no. 1, pp. 45–51

47   Ruth Winter, "Your Health and Your Dreams," *Family Circle,* July 1966.

47   Irwin Feinberg, M.D., et al., "Patterns of Sleep Over a Lifetime," Mental Health Programs Report 2, February 1968, p. 167, National Institutes of Health.

47   Jo Thomas, "Normal Behavior Inaccurately Labeled Senile," *Miami Herald,* February 20, 1972.

49   "Noise Studies Confirm Hazard to Animals and Man," *Medical Tribune,* January 28, 1970, p. 24.

49   Jacek Szabran, "Psychological Studies of Aging Pilots," *Aerospace Medicine,* May 1969, pp. 543–53.

49   Ruth Winter, "How Intense Are Your Senses," *Family Circle,* August 1967.

50   "On the Brains and Minds of Older Patients," *Medical World News,* March 19, 1971, pp. 78–80.

50   Carl Eisdorfer, Ph.D., M.D., "Psychological Aspects of Learning in the Aged–A Tentative Theory," national conference, Manpower Training and the Older Workers, January 17–19, 1966, Washington, D.C.

51   Wilder Penfield, M.D., *Epilepsy and the Functional Anatomy of the Human Brain,* Little, Brown, Boston, 1954.

51,52   Enjar J. Fjerdingstad, Ph.D., "Further Studies of Chemical Transfer of Learned Behavior in the Goldfish," presented at the American Association for the Advancement of Science, December 30, 1970, Chicago.

52,53   "Mechanisms of Memory," *Lancet,* January 18, 1969, 1:40.

52   Georges Unger, M.D., "Chemical Transfer of Passive Avoidance," presented to the Federation of American Societies for Experimental Biology, Atlantic City, April 17, 1969, and United Press International article, January 22, 1971.

52,53   Eleanor A. Jacobs, M.D., S. Mouchly Small, M.D., and Peter Winters, M.D., "Hyperbaric Oxygen in Treatment of Senility," presented at the American Psychological Association meeting, Washington, D.C., May 1970; and Joan Lynn Arehart, "Retaining Memory in Older People," *Science News,* March 18, 1972, vol. 101, p. 3.

53   D. E. Cameron, "Recent Advances in Biological Psychiatry," *Medical Tribune,* 1967, 9:1.

53   A. S. Kulkarni, Ph.D., "Magnesium Pemoline: Specificity of Effects on Instrumental Avoidance Learning," *Behavioral Science,* 1970.

53   John Nowlin, Ph.D., interview with author, Durham, North Carolina, January 18, 1971.

53   Henry Altschuler, Ph.D., Charles Harris, M.D., and Samuel Granick, Ph.D., "Survival Linked with Retention of Intellectual, Social Stability,"

presented at the International Congress of Gerontology, Washington, D.C., 1970.

54   Paul Gordon, Ph.D., "Chemical Basis for Anti-viral Action," presented to the Federation of American Societies for Experimental Biology, April 13, 1971, Chicago; Paul Gordon, "Molecular Approaches to the Drug Enhancement of Deteriorated Functioning in the Aged," *Advances in Gerontological Research*, New York, Academic Press, 1971, vol. 3.

54   "Anti-coagulant Therapy May Aid Senile Patients," *Journal of the American Medical Association.* May 22, 1972, vol. 220, no. 8, p. 1065.

54   M. L. Mitra, "Senility Yields to Vitamin Therapy," *Journal of the American Geriatrics Society*, May 1971.

54   Ward C. Halstead, M.D., "Biological Intelligence and Differential Aging," in *Aging—A Current Appraisal*, I. L. Webber, editor, Gainesville, University of Florida Press, 1956, pp. 63–75.

55   Ewald Busse, M.D., interview with author, January 13, 1971,, Durham, North Carolina.

55   Bernard M. Patten, M.D., *Archives of Neurology*, January 1972.

56   Nathan Shock, Ph.D., "Age with a Future," *The Gerontologist*, Autumn 1968, vol. 8, no. 3, pp. 147–52.

Chapter 6

57   "How Strong Is the Skin?" *Medical World News*, October 2, 1970.

58,59   *Working with Older People: The Practitioner and the Elderly*, U.S. Department of Health, Education and Welfare, March 1969, pp. 12–13.

60   Messam Fikry, M.D., "The Aging Cell: Aging and Death as Aspects of Growth and Development: Natural Phenomena Controlled by Genetic Factors," *American Geriatrics Society Journal*, November 1969, vol. 17, no. 11, pp. 1044–54.

60,61   "The Aging Skin," Department of Health, Education and Welfare, *American Medical Association Bulletin*, 9801-711G:1070-5M, Chicago, 1970.

61,62   Albert Kligman, M.D., "Early Destructive Effect of Sunlight on Human Skin," *Journal of the American Medical Association*, December 29, 1969, vol. 210, no. 13, pp. 2377–80.

61,62   "The Sun and Your Skin," Department of Health Education, American Medical Association, Chicago, 1970.

63   Harry W. Daniell, M.D., "Smokers Wrinkles," *Annals of Internal Medicine*, December 1971, 75: 873–80.

63   Marvin Chernosky, M.D., "Dry Skin and Its Consequences," *Journal of the American Medical Women's Association, March* 1972, vol. 27, no. 4, pp. 133–45.

64   Marjorie Bauer, M.D., "Cosmetic Quackery," presented to the Fourth National Congress on Health Quackery, October 2, 1968, Chicago.

64   Howard Behrman, M.D., interview with author, April 20, 1971, New York.

64   Irwin Lubowe, M.D., "Treatment of the Aging Skin," *Geriatrics Digest*, vol. 7, pp. 7–13.

65,66,69   D. McCullagh Mayer, M.D., interview with author, May 9, 1969, Atlantic City.

67,68   Thomas J. Barker, Jr., M.D., "Ten Year Report on Chemical Face Peel," presented to the American College of Surgeons convention, 1972.

70,71   "Sale of Health and Beauty Aids in Drug Stores, Grocery Stores and Other Outlets," *Drug Trade News*, 1968.

70,71   Veronica Conley, "Gray Hair," *Today's Health*, October 1953.

72   Martin Wortzel, M.D., interview with author, May 1969, Millburn, New Jersey.

72   James Hamilton, Ph.D., personal communication with author, March–April 1971.

72,73   Howard Behrman, M.D., "Scalp in Health," New York: Mosby, 1952.

73,74   "The Aging Skin," American Medical Association information sheet, April 8, 1969.

Chapter 7

76   Nathan Shock, Ph.D., interview with author, March 3, 1971.

76   "Live Longer and Like It," a science feature article prepared by the American Medical Association's Department of Science News, 1968.

76   H. Bismark and D. Medzinischen, Klink-Halle, Universitats, East Germany, "Adiposity as a Pacemaking and Common Factor of Polymor-

bidity During Old Age," A6800099, Adult Development and Aging Abstracts, 1968, no. 1, U.S. Department of Health, Education and Welfare.

76 Clive McCay, Ph.D., G. Sperling, and L. L. Barnes, "Growth, Aging, Chronic Diseases and Life Span in Rats," *Archives of Biochemistry*, 1943, 2:469.

77,78 Charles Barrow, Ph.D., interview with author, March 3, 1971, Baltimore.

78,79 "Scientists Find Age of Maturity in Children Has Steadily Declined in Last 300 Years," in *The New York Times*, January 24, 1971.

78,79 U.S. Public Health Service Survey, 1971.

79,80 Myron Winick, M.D., and A. Noble, *Developmental Biology*, 1965, 12:451; *Journal of Nutrition*, 1966, 89:300.

80 S. Hejda, Institute für Ernährungs Forschung, Czechoslovakia, "Nutrition Conditions During Childhood in Long-Lived Persons," A6900098, Adult Development and Aging Abstracts of the National Institute of Child Health and Human Development, 1969, no. 4.

80 K. H. Mann, M.D., interview with author, June 1972, New York, and author's research, Israel, July–August 1971.

81,82,83, Denham Harmon, M.D., Ph.D.,
84 interview with author, March 16, 1971, New York.

83 "Cancer Deaths Found Higher in Trial of Polyunsaturates," *Medical Tribune*, December 7, 1970.

84 P. Gyorgy et al., *Pediatrics*, 1958, 21: 673.

84,85 Max Horwitt, Ph.D., "Vitamin E in Human Nutrition: An Interpretive Review," *Borden's Review of Nutrition Research*, January, March 1961, vol. 22, no. 1.

84,85 A. L. Tappel, Ph.D., "Lipid Peroxidation Damage to Cell Components," presented to the Federation of American Societies for Experimental Biology's Fifth Annual Meeting, April 16, 1970.

84,85 "Vitamin E Background Information," Vitamin Information Bureau, 575 Lexington Avenue, N.Y. 10022.

84,85 Kurt Haeger, M.D., "The Treatment of Peripheral Occlusive Disease with a-Tocopherol, as Compared With Vasodialator Agents and Antiprothrombin (Dicumerol)," *Vascular Diseases*, December 1968, vol. 5, no. 4, pp. 199–212; Campbell Moses, M.D., medical director, American Heart Association, interview with author, June 1970, New York.

84,85 Evan Shute, M.D., Letters to Editor, *Science News*, January 15, 1972, and personal communication with author, April 1972.

86 "Zinc: Human Nutrition and Metabolic Effects," *Annals of Internal Medicine*, 1970, 73: 631–36, and "A Zinc Backgrounder," Vitamin Information Bureau, New York, 1971.

86 "Exploring Nickel Deficiency," Agricultural Research, U.S. Department of Agriculture, October 1970, pp. 6–7.

86 "Chromium May Help Solve Old-Age Health Problems," U.S. Department of Agriculture Report, Washington, D.C., December 3, 1971.

86,87 Bill Kovach, "Pollution by Toxic Metals Called Most Harmful," *The New York Times*, September 1, 1970.

87 Kathy Mahan, "Does Low Calcium Intake Cause Osteoporosis," *Journal of the American Medical Association*, October 11, 1971, vol. 218, no. 2, p. 263.

87 "Soft Water, Hard Arteries," *Medical Tribune* editorial, January 1971, and "Lithium in Water Could Lower Rate of Heart Disease," *Journal of the American Medical Association*, December 7, 1970, vol. 214, no. 10, p. 1789.

87 "United States Department of Agriculture Scientists Report on Mineral Research," Washington, D.C., September 21, 1970.

88–91 American Medical Association literature and U.S. Department of Agriculture literature.

Chapter 8

94 "Exercisers and Researchers at Y Here Have Heart in Mind," *The New York Times*, March 14, 1971, p. 48; Joseph B. Wolfe, M.D. "Physical Activity in the Prevention and Treatment of Atherosclerosis and Its Complications," presented to the Scientific Regional Conference of the American College of Sports Medicine, October 27, 1963, Norristown, Pennsylvania.

94,96 A. H. Ishmail, John Young of Purdue University, paper presented March 27, 1972, Houston, Texas, before the American Association for Health, Physical Education and Recreation.

94 "Good News for Men Over 30," *Medical World News*, February 26, 1971, p. 13.

94 University of California *News*, November 3, 1970.

94 "Fitness Tests Reveal Young Are in Worse Shape Than Their Elders," Loma Linda University *News*, December 8, 1970.

94 C. L. Donaldson, et al., "Effects of Prolonged Bed Rest on Bone Mineral," *Metabolism*, December 1970, 19: 1071–84.

95 Ralph S. Paffenbarger, Jr., M.D., et. al., "Characteristics of Longshoremen Related to Fatal Coronary Heart Disease and Stroke," *American Journal of Public Health*, July 1971, vol. 61, no. 7, pp. 1962–70.

96 Ruth Winter, "Exercise Adds Bounce During Those Later Years," *Newark Sunday Star-Ledger* article about Cincinnati heart specialist Robert S. Green, M.D., speech before the American Medical Association, April 30, 1967.

96 Paul Dudley White, M.D., "The Role of Exercise in the Aging," *Health Aspects of Aging*, American Medical Association booklet, Chicago, 1965.

96 "Exercise Lack Seen to Cause Disability in Normal Women," *Medical Tribune*, Monday, March 2, 1970.

97 Nathan Shock, Ph.D., "Physical Activity and the Rage of Aging," *Canadian Medical Association Journal*, March 25, 1967, 96: 836–40; Nathan Shock, Ph.D., "The Physiology of Aging," *Scientific American*, January 1962, pp. 2–10, and interview with author, March 3, 1971, Baltimore.

98,99 Earl W. Ferguson, et al., "Exercise, Blood Coagulation and Fibrinolytic Activity," presented at the Federation of American Societies for Experimental Biology, April 18, 1969, Atlantic City.

99 L. A. Carlson, et al., "Effect of Training with Exercise on Plasma and Tissue Lipid Levels of Aging Rats," *Gerontologia*, January 1969, pp. 14–23.

Dr. Ashok K. Bhan and Dr. James Scheuer, "Exercise and

ATPase," presented before the 44th annual scientific session of the American Heart Association, November 14, 1971, Anaheim, California.

99,100 "Methods of Exercise Studied in Men," *Medical Tribune*, November 10, 1971, pp. 27–54.

99,100 Paul Dudley White, M.D., *Journal of the American Medical Association*, 1958, vol. 167, no. 6, p. 711.

104 *Osteoarthritis: A Handbook for Patients*, The Arthritis Foundation, 1212 Avenue of the Americas, New York 10036, 1967.

104 Albert Ferguson, Jr., M.D., "The Age of Repair," *Geriatrics Medical World News Annual*, 1971, pp. 34–38.

106,107 "Seventy-Five-Year-Old Woman Conquers 14,495-foot Mt. Whitney," Loma Linda news release, August 23, 1971. Loma Linda, California.

107,108, *Exercise and Health: A Point of View*, American Medical Association booklet, 1970.

108,109 The Committee on Exercise and Physical Fitness of the American Medical Association and the President's Council on Physical Fitness and Sports Report, *Journal of the American Medical Association*, February 14, 1972.

Chapter 9

110 Eric Pfeiffer, M.D., "Sex and Aging," *Medical Aspects of Human Sexuality*, October 1972, pp. 17–21.

110 "Various Sexual Problems Blamed for Male Infertility," Medical News Section, *Journal of the American Medical Association*, May 8, 1972, vol. 220, no. 6. p. 780.

110,116 Robert L. Rown, M.D., "Love at All Seasons Means the Aged Too," *Modern Medicine*, May 1, 1972, pp. 29–30.

110,116 "Understanding Urged of Forms of Sexual Expression by Aged," *Roche Report: Frontiers of Clinical Psychiatry*, October 1, 1970.

112,113 Howard D. Weiss, M.D., Mechanism of Erection," *Medical Aspects of Human Sexuality*, February 1973, pp. 28–44.

114 Hans Zinsser, M.D., "Time's Effect on the Prostate," *Medical World News Geriatrics*, 1972, pp. 19–20.

114 C. David Cawood, M.D., "Petting and Prostatic Engorge-

ment," *Medical Aspects of Human Sexuality,* November 1967, pp. 204–15.

116 Arnold A. Lazarus, Ph.D., "Psychological Causes of Impotence," *Sexual Behavior,* September 1972, pp. 39–44.

118,119 Eleanor B. Rodgerson, M.D., "Beyond the Menopause," *Medical World News Geriatrics,* 1972, pp. 30–31.

120 Marvin G. Drellich, M.D., "Sex After Hysterectomy," *Medical Aspects of Human Sexuality,* November 1967, pp. 146–54.

Chapter 10

121 Philip Enterline and Dr. William Stewart, Public Health Reports, September 1956, United States Public Health Service.

122 "Mortality in Selected Countries, 1954–55 and 1964–65," Metropolitan Life *Statistical Bulletin,* February 1971.

122 "Is Longevity Linked to Loot, Learning, Libido?" *Journal of the American Medical Association,* September 22, 1969, vol. 209, no. 12, p. 1827.

123 "Chronic Ills: Rise Linked to Pollution," *Medical Tribune,* January 13, 1971, p. 1.

123,124 James Watson, Ph.D., interview with author, January 18, 1971, New York.

123,124 Samuel S. Epstein, M.D., "Chemical Mutagens in the Environment," American Association for Cancer Research, March 23, 1969, San Francisco.

124 Morris Pollard, Ph.D., interview with author, April 22, 1971, Indiana; Morris Pollard, Ph.D., and Mashiro Kajima, "Lesions in Aged Germ Free Wistar Rats," The American Association for Laboratory Animal Science, November 5, 1971, Chicago.

125 Wayne Smith, planning office, UCLA at Los Angeles, "Factors Associated with Age and Specific Death Rates," *Journal of Public Health,* 1968, 58 (10), 1937–49.

125 "Twelve Pancreatitis Cases in a Town in Maryland Blamed on Air Pollution," *Medical Tribune,* February 10, 1971, p. 3.

125 Warren Winklestein, Jr., and M. L. Gag, "Suspended Particulate Air Pollution," *Archives of Environmental Health,* January 1971, vol. 22, pp. 174–77.

125 Bertram Carnow, M.D., et al., "The Role of Air Pollution in Chronic Obstructive Pulmonary Disease," *Journal of the American Medical Association,* November 2, 1970, vol. 214, pp. 894–99.

125 "Environmental Quality," the first annual report of the Council on Environmental Quality, August 1970, Washington, D.C.

126 Ruth Winter, "Pollutants Inside the Home," *World Book Science Service,* December 7, 1969.

128 "Radiation Deaths: Estimate Tripled in Controversy," *Medical Tribune,* April 14, 1971.

129 U.S. Department of Health, Education and Welfare announcement, November 2, 1967, and personal communication with Harold J. Perkins, Ph.D., April 1971.

129 "Cancer Risk in the Chem Lab?" *Medical World News,* May 8, 1970, p. 29.

129 "Asbestos: The Need for and Feasibility of Air Pollution Controls," National Research Council's Committee on Biologic Effects of Atmospheric Pollutants, National Academy of Sciences, 2101 Constitution Avenue N.W., Washington, D.C. 20418, October 8, 1971.

129,130 Jules V. Quint, B.S., and Bianca Cody, M.A., "Pre-eminence and Mortality: Longevity of Prominent Men," *American Journal of Public Health,* June 1970, vol. 60, no. 6, pp. 1118–24.

129,130 "Longevity of Members of Congress," Metropolitan Life *Statistical Bulletin,* December 1970.

129,135 J. L. Haybrittle, "Cigarette Smoking and Life Expectancy," *British Journal of Preventive and Social Medicine,* April 1966, vol. 20, pp. 101–4.

130 Hans Selye, Ph.D., *The Stress of Life,* McGraw-Hill, New York, 1956.

130 James Naiman, M.D., *Journal of Geriatric Psychiatry,* November 1968, pp. 102–13.

131 James Nix, M.D., and Con Fecher, M.D., "The Study of the Cause of Death of Nuns," 1963–1970, and personal communication with authors, May 5, 1971.

131 *The Social Sciences and Human Biology,* Russell Sage Foundation, 1968–1969, p. 19.

131 George Comstock, M.D., De-

partment of Epidemiology, Johns Hopkins University, NIH Report, October 15, 1971.

131 R. Sh. Alikishiyev, "Basic Factors in Longevity in Daghestan and Prolongation of Life," second conference on gerontology and geriatrics, Moscow, 1960 (translation by U.S. Department of Health, Education and Welfare, Public Health Service publication, no. 884.

132 David A. Andelman, "Andes Evidence Indicts Cholesterol," *The New York Times,* April 22, 1971, p. 43.

133 Eric Pfeiffer, M.D., "Survival in Old Age: Physical, Psychological and Social Correlates of Longevity," *Journal of the American Geriatrics Society,* April 1970, vol. 28, no. 4, pp. 273–85.

133 Erdman Palmore, Ph.D., "Physical, Mental and Social Factors in Predicting Longevity," *The Gerontologist,* Summer 1969, pp. 103–8, and interview with author, January 13, 1971, Durham, North Carolina.

134,135 "Want to Live a Long Life? Seek Goals Firmly But Gently," press release by the Colorado Medical Society, June 22, 1967, Denver.

135 Murray Parkes, B. Benjamin, and R. Fitzgerald, "Broken Heart: A Statistical Study of Increased Mortality Among Widowers," *British Medical Journal,* January 1969, pp. 740–43.

Postscript

136 Benjamin Schloss, Ph.D., interview with author, November 11, 1970, New York.

137 "Health Characteristics of the Elderly," Metropolitan Life *Statistical Bulletin,* August 1968.

137 Hearings of the Special Committee on Aging, U.S. Senate, "Adequacy of Services for Older Workers," July 24, 25, and 29, 1968, Washington, D.C.

137 Robert Garber, Ph.D., of Roher, Hibler and Replogle, a national firm of consulting psychologists, interview with author, May 1969, New York.

137 Allen Bernard, "The Tragic Plight of the Aging Physician," *Medical Opinion,* January 1972.

137,138 Ewald Busse, M.D., "The Modern Challenge of Three Score Years and Ten,' symposium, "Man—the Mature Years and Beyond," April 16, 1969, Chicago.

139 Joseph W. Still, M.D., testimony on Hearts of the Special Committee on Aging, op. cit.; David K. Shipler, "City Pension Costs Snowballing," *The New York Times,* March 15, 1971, p. 1.

140 Gerald Feinberg, Ph.D., "Can We and Should We Do Anything to Prolong Youth?" New York Public Library Forum, January 11, 1971.

140 Cicero's "De Senectute."

141 Nathan Shock, Ph.D., interview with author, March 3, 1971, Baltimore.

141 Ewald Busse, M.D., interview with author, January 13, 1971, Durham, North Carolina.

141 Robert Browning, "Rabbi Ben Ezra."

Index